Reviews of *Diagnosis and Treatment of Cl Syndrome, Myalgic Encephalitis and Long*

Dr Myhill has written an extraordinary book. She is the number one authority on CFS in the UK. Whereas many doctors dismiss the condition, she explains what it is, what has gone wrong in the body, using appropriate tests that are not done by mainstream medicine, and tells people what they can do about it. Whereas mainstream medicine only uses drugs to deal with a particular symptom, Dr Myhill explains the reasons 'Why'. In my opinion, you will never cure anything unless you understand and deal with the why.

Dr P J Kingsley MB BS, MRCS, LRCP, FAAEM, DA, DObst, RCOG

This book is logical and evidence-based but is still an easy read. Dr Myhill has made the mitochondrial story clear for the non-expert. It makes essential reading for family members or friends of CFS sufferers. This book will help these patients to obtain understanding and effective management from their physicians.

Dr Sybil Birtwistle MB ChB, DObst, RCOG, DCH, Post Graduate Tutor, British Society for Environmental Medicine

This book is an invaluable tool to recover from fatigue-related disorders for patients and practitioners alike! It is based on years of clinical experience, backed by research; written in a clear, concise way with lots of practical instructions – and from what I can see using these methods in my practice: it works!

Dr Franziska Meuschel MD, PhD, ND, LFhom

The first edition of this book became a key reference that was readable and upbeat, full of information explaining complex issues of cell biology together with practical tips. ... Many important tests are explained in detail together with their role in a person's recovery plan. The folly of the mainstream approach to ME is exposed and is truly shocking. The style is flowing; the evidence is poignant and the references are meticulously made, yet easy to follow. Dr Myhill has opened the minds of thousands of ME sufferers, and their carers, as to how to seize control of their health in an era when evidence is mounting that the causes of many chronic conditions can be traced to our lifestyles and environment.

Dr Apelles Econs MRCS, LRCP, Allergist

Brilliant! This book offers the most complete, logical, practical and optimistic guide for people trying to recover from CFS that I am aware of. If every doctor could also take its contents on board, the management of CFS would be revolutionised.

Dr Charles Forsyth MB BS, FFHom

Over the years, working as a General Practitioner, I have recommended Dr Myhill's work to hundreds of patients. Her approach combines an in-depth understanding of human physiology with years of practical experience, and the use of cutting-edge laboratory testing, to diagnose and treat the root causes of complex chronic diseases. Written with humour and compassion, Dr Myhill has put together a simple step-by-step guide for patients, to take back control of their own health and start their journey to recovery. I am delighted that I can now recommend this book to every patient.

Dr Jens Rohrbeck MD (Dr med), MPhil, GP and Functional Medicine Physician

This book is a 'must have' for everyone suffering from CFS (and their doctors). It explains all the different aspects of this complex condition, and details ways that each patient can contribute to their own recovery. Dr Myhill has tirelessly dedicated much of her career to improving the quality of life of CFS patients for whom conventional approaches (antidepressants, cognitive behavioural therapy and graded exercise) have not been enough. Her commitment, genius and sense of humour come across wonderfully in these pages, encouraging and supporting those with this terrible condition not to give up.

Dr Nicola Hembry BSc, MB BS, MSB, PGDip

The brilliant work of John McLaren-Howard, Sarah Myhill and Norman Booth reveals that CFS/ME is due to mitochondrial dysfunction. This discovery revolutionizes the world's understanding of CFS and how to investigate and treat the biochemical abnormalities. Dr Myhill's book has never been more needed. ... The epidemic of CFS, like breast cancer, has increased since contraceptive hormone and HRT use became widespread. Mitochondrial dysfunction has many causes, including toxic DNA adducts, but avoiding progestin and oestrogen use is vitally important for recovery from CFS.

Dr Ellen Grant MB ChB, DObst, RCOG

Dr Myhill breaks new ground in her approach to chronic fatigue syndrome and demonstrates clearly, with compelling scientific evidence, that this condition is not psychological but has treatable physical causes. She gives detailed guidance on practical ecological measures that need to be followed to effect recovery. This is a book which should cause many doctors and health professionals to radically revise their understanding of CFS and gives sufferers real encouragement and hope for their future health.

Dr John Meldrum MB ChB, MRCGP, DA, DCH, DObst RCOG, HTD

What really struck me about this book is the degree to which it allows people with CFS to be in charge of their own recovery, and to have the confidence, through the authority of the author, to know what to ask for from health professionals. It explains with real clarity the complex biochemical processes underlying chronic disease and CFS, and the link with allergies, diet, micro-organisms and aspects of the Western lifestyle. There is a detailed and clear discussion of the tests available, how to interpret them, and what to do to get better. All this without ignoring the importance of good lifestyle habits, psychological health and the right kind of exercise. A fantastic book for all health professionals too.

Dr Dee Marshall MB BS, MFHom, WellnessMedical, London, UK

Dr Myhill's wonderful book presents the clearest and most helpful information I have ever read on what chronic fatigue syndrome actually is and what the many possible causes of it are. This is the ***only book*** *that I've found that presents a comprehensive approach for assessing the underlying causes of CFS and treating them in a way that may be tailored for the individual patient. Understanding how mitochondrial failure can arise, why mitochondrial function problems are often a major factor in CFS and the approaches for restoring good mitochondrial function should form part of all medical training. Dr Myhill's book should be a standard text in all medical schools as well as being essential reading for all CFS patients and their doctors. It is easy to read, laden with information and shows practical ways of actually assessing and treating CFS. Loved it!*

Paul Robinson BSc (Hons), author of *Recovering with T3* and *The CT3M Handbook*

Drawing on decades of clinical experience, and unparalleled success in restoring health, hope and energy to thousands of CFS patients, Dr Myhill brings solid scientific evidence together with biological common sense to explain how to recover from this ghastly and increasingly common illness. She describes the underlying cellular mechanisms in a way that everyone can understand, demonstrating simply the physiological basis of low energy production in CFS. This is an aspect that is largely ignored by most current approaches to CFS, but Dr Myhill shows clearly that CFS is in your mitochondria, not in your mind! This book is an invaluable step-by-step guide to recovery, for patient and physician alike. I would not be without a copy in my clinic!

Dr Jenny Goodman MA, MB ChB

SM: I dedicate this book to Dr John McLaren-Howard and Professor Norman Booth. John's brilliance in developing mitochondrial function tests demonstrated that patients with fatigues have real pathology. He showed they were mitochondriacs not hypochondriacs. Norman put this on the world stage by getting this work published with his usual academic rigour. A big thank you from patients and physicians alike!

CR: Once again it has been an absolute pleasure and privilege to work with Sarah. I dedicate this book to my two children, Gina and Conor. They have never known me without ME; I hope that one day they will. In any case, one thing is for sure; I have learnt more from them than they have from me. They are my pride and joy and I have been inspired by them more than they will ever know. Here is their wisdom:

- Gina Hull – 'Always be a little kinder than necessary' (J M Barrie (9 May 1860 – 19 June 1937))
- Conor Robinson – 'At the end of the game, the king and the pawn are placed in the same box' (Old Italian Proverb)

THIRD EDITION

Diagnosis and Treatment of CHRONIC FATIGUE SYNDROME, MYALGIC ENCEPHALITIS AND LONG-COVID

it's mitochondria, not hypochondria

DR SARAH MYHILL AND CRAIG ROBINSON

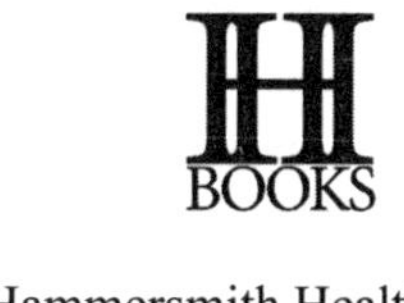

Hammersmith Health Books
London, UK

First published in 2024 by Hammersmith Health Books
– an imprint of Hammersmith Books Limited
4/4A Bloomsbury Square, London WC1A 2RP, UK
www.hammersmithbooks.co.uk

The information contained in this book is for educational purposes only. It is the result of the study and the experience of the authors. Whilst the information and advice offered are believed to be true and accurate at the time of going to press, neither the authors nor the publisher can accept any legal responsibility or liability for any errors or omissions that may have been made or for any adverse effects which may occur as a result of following the recommendations given herein. Always consult a qualified medical practitioner if you have any concerns regarding your health.
British Library Cataloguing in Publication Data: A CIP record of this book is available from the British Library.

Print ISBN 978-1-78161-254-5
Ebook ISBN 978-1-78161-255-2

Commissioning editor: Georgina Bentliff
Designed and typeset by: Julie Bennett of Bespoke Publishing Limited
Cover illustrations: Christopher Hoare
Cover design by: Julie Bennett of Bespoke Publishing Limited
Index: Dr Laurence Errington
Production: Deborah Wehner of Moatvale Press, UK
Printed and bound by: TJ Books Ltd, Cornwall, UK

Contents

About the Authors

Dr Sarah Myhill MB BS qualified in medicine (with Honours) from Middlesex Hospital Medical School in 1981 and has since focused tirelessly on identifying and treating the underlying causes of health problems, especially the 'diseases of civilisation' with which we are beset in the West. She has worked in the NHS and independent practice and for 17 years was the Honorary Secretary of the British Society for Ecological Medicine, which focuses on the causes of disease and treating through diet, supplements and avoiding toxic stress. She helps to run and lectures at the Society's training courses and also lectures regularly on organophosphate poisoning, the problems of silicone, and chronic fatigue syndrome. She is also Medical Director of UK Medical Freedom Alliance, Medical Director of CNM, and has been awarded an Honorary Diploma in Naturopathic Medicine in recognition of her outstanding contribution to the field of Natural Medicine. Visit her website at www.drmyhill.co.uk

Craig Robinson MA took a first in Mathematics at Oxford University in 1985. He then joined Price Waterhouse and qualified as a Chartered Accountant in 1988, after which he worked as a lecturer in the private sector, and also in the City of London, primarily in Financial Sector Regulation roles. Craig first met Sarah in 2001, as a patient for the treatment of his ME and since then they have developed a professional working relationship, where he helps with the maintenance of www.drmyhill.co.uk, the moderating of Dr Myhill's Facebook groups and other ad hoc projects, as well as with the editing and writing of her books.

Preface

This third edition of *Diagnosis and Treatment of Chronic Fatigue Syndrome, Myalgic Encephalitis and Long Covid* is written on a 'need-to-know' basis, as follows:

	What you need to know	**What you need to do**
Introduction	This book is written on the need-to-know principle	Take a leap of faith and just do it
Chapter 1	The road map for recovery	The overall strategy: • Improve energy delivery • Plug the immunological holes in the energy bucket • Plug the emotional holes
Chapter 2	Chronic fatigue syndrome: the symptoms of poor energy delivery	Use symptoms to discern mechanisms…
Chapter 3	Overview of the mechanisms of poor energy delivery and how to fix them	…because that has obvious implications for how they are managed
Chapter 4	First do the PK diet, then sort out the upper fermenting gut then take the Basic Package of supplements	Sort out the fuel in the tank
Chapter 5	The mitochondrial engines	Take the supplements Start to detox
Chapter 6	Oxygen	Breathe properly
Chapter 7	The thyroid accelerator pedal and the adrenal gearbox	How to balance up essential hormones

	What you need to know	What you need to do
Chapter 8	Sleep – when healing and repair take place	Sleep is as vital as diet and pacing
Chapter 9	Pacing and the right sort of exercise	Yes, it is boring but you will recover more quickly
Chapter 10	Myalgic encephalitis and long Covid – the symptoms of inflammation	Use symptoms to discern mechanisms…
Chapter 11	Overview of the mechanisms of inflammation and how to fix them	…because that has obvious implications for how they are managed
Chapter 12	Allergy and autoimmunity	How to recognise and deal with these
Chapter 13	The general approach to reducing inflammation	How to plug these immunological holes
Chapter 14	Detoxing to reduce the toxic load of metals, pesticides, volatile organic compounds, prescription drugs, mycotoxins and more	Toxins increase the biochemical friction – How to avoid and reduce the endogenous load
Chapter 15	The general approach to treating chronic infection – reduce the infectious load	We all carry infections – how to start minimising that burden
Chapter 16	DMSO (dimethylsulphoxide)	A wonderful multitasking tool
Chapter 17	Methylene blue for many chronic infections	Reduce the total infectious load
Chapter 18	Photodynamic therapy – using light to kill infections	Ditto
Chapter 19	Reprogramming the immune system with micro-immunotherapy	Train the immune system to focus its fire and behave itself
Chapter 20	Reducing the infectious load with specific antimicrobials	Which tests to do to identify microbes
Chapter 21	Plugging the emotional holes in the energy bucket	Avoid doctors Sleep, love, pets, money, humour, meditation, connecting with others
Chapter 22	The pattern of recovery	Just do it

	What you need to know	**What you need to do**
Chapter 23	The politics of CFS and ME – the name, the shame and the blame	How we humans are poisoning the World and destroying ourselves in the process – The early symptoms of this are CFS and ME
Appendix 1	Groundhog Basic	What we should all be doing all the time to prevent disease and live to our full potential
Appendix 1	Groundhog Acute	What we should all do at the first hint of any acute infection
Appendix 1	Groundhog Chronic	What we should all be doing all the time as we become chronically ill or aged
Appendix 2	Diet, detox and die off (DDD) reactions	You may get worse, initially, in response to a healing intervention, but things will get better
Appendix 3	Commonly used tests and how to interpret them	Important clues are often missed – look at the actual figures and reference ranges
Appendix 4	How to access benefits	Get what you're entitled to
Appendix 5	The Bell CFS ability scale	How sick are you?

The 'need-to-know' principle or basis is technically a term used by Governments, and often their Armed Forces, to denote situations where people are told the bare minimum to carry out their duties – i.e., up to their respective security clearance levels only. The Battle of Normandy in 1944 is a classic example of this. Many thousands of military personnel were involved in planning the invasion, but only a small number of them knew the entire plans of the operation; the rest only knew the data needed to complete their small part of the plan.

In the context of this book, the 'need-to-know' basis is not intended to obscure important details from the reader but rather to keep the size of the book to a minimum whilst at the same time conveying all that is needed to be known and, hopefully at the same time, keeping you, dear reader, entertained at regular intervals throughout. Learning happens better if enjoyment is involved. In essence, the authors are aware that many readers are likely to be cognitively challenged and so this 'need-to-know' basis is the best format, and this is also why we have included short chapter summaries.

If you *do* wish to know more, then my 500+ page website, www.drmyhill.co.uk, and our books *Ecological Medicine*, *The Infection Game* and *Paleo-ketogenic: The Why and the How* supply most of the answers, but for the time being, let us proceed as stated, safe in the knowledge that Douglas Adams agrees with us when he wrote in *The Hitchhikers Guide to the Galaxy* that he wished to be protected from things he didn't need to know. Indeed, he wished protection from even knowing that there were things that he didn't need to know!

Key terminology

The following abbreviations are used in this book:

CFS – chronic fatigue syndrome

ME – myalgic encepahalitis

LC – long Covid

What these terms actually mean is detailed in Chapters 2 and 10, but in brief:

- Chronic fatigue syndrome (CFS) is characterised by poor energy delivery mechanisms.
- Myalgic encephalitis (ME) is characterised by poor energy delivery mechanisms *and* inflammation.
- Long Covid is ME which follows acute Covid infection and/or Covid-19 mRNA gene therapy 'vaccines'.

Poor energy delivery is caused by poor diet and gut function, poor breathing, poor sleep, mitochondrial failure and poor adrenal and thyroid function.

Inflammation occurs when the immune system is activated. The immune system is activated in allergy, chronic infection and autoimmunity.

Stylistic note: Use of the first-person singular in this book refers to me, Dr Sarah Myhill. One can assume that the medicine, biochemistry and opinions are mine, as edited by Craig Robinson, and that the classical and mathematical references are Craig's.

Introduction

This book details the practical reality of recovering from chronic fatigue syndrome (CFS), myalgic-encephalitis (ME) and long Covid (LC). I have been working with sufferers of these conditions since 1981, in the cases of CFS and ME, when I qualified as a doctor, and for the last three years in the case of LC. The early stages of the recovery journey I know, from that experience, are non-negotiable and essential. Many will recover simply by implementing these early stages. Some of the later stages are still on trial, but biologically plausible, safe and eminently doable. Recovery is like building a house – you have to start with the foundation stones of diet, gut function and micronutrients, and then build on that. It is not a case of either/or; to restore health you have to do the whole shooting match.

The Third Little Pig in the well-known fairytale* knew this well, when he built his house from brick, rather than straw or sticks. It took longer to build but it (and I ad-lib a little here) had good foundations and so the Big Bad Wolf could not blow it down. Do take the time and effort to put in place the important foundations for your recovery – they will serve you well.

I am painfully aware that many with CFS, ME and LC lack the energy and resources and may be dismayed by the prospect of the journey to wellness. For that reason, in this

**The Three Little Pigs* is a fable that dates back in printed form to 1840, but is thought to be much older than that and, in one of its earliest forms, is set on Dartmoor with three pixies and a fox.

book I have tried to describe the route to recovery that is the shortest, quickest and most frictionless. I have tried to give the Why in sufficient detail to provide sufferers with the intellectual imperative to make the necessary changes, but not to bog them down in detail. I then move on to the How. Again, I have consciously eschewed some of the detail so that readers do not lose the logical progression and maintain the momentum for recovery. I only include the absolute basic interventions which are universally necessary. I have learned this from over four decades of trial and error. Throughout, I direct readers to my other books should they wish for more detail, but it is not necessary to purchase these for most to recover. As already emphasised in the Contents section, this book is written on the need-to-know principle.

I start with the 'Rules of the Game' and move on the 'Tools of the Trade'. These tools need to be safe, multi-tasking, easy to implement and available to all because most of my patients are unable to work and cannot afford expensive treatments. They are not RBs[†]; they are PBs. (Hereinafter in this book, 'RB' shall refer to 'Rich Bastard' and 'PB' shall refer to 'Poor Bastard'. Isn't the English language wonderful? In RB, the 'B' elicits disdain in the reader, whereas in PB, it evokes sympathy, even empathy!)

These Tools of the Trade are not just for those with CFS, ME and LC. They are also the starting point to prevent and treat all diseases of Westerners – degeneration, dementia, cancer and heart disease. It means I can tell my patients with complete confidence that, with all these regimes in place, they will also live to their full potential in terms of quality and quantity of life. Indeed, fatigue is often an early warning symptom of such disease, a symptom for which conventional medicine has little to offer with its symptom-suppressing prescription drugs. By suppressing symptoms, the warning signs are missed and the underlying pathology is accelerated.

We do not have enough therapists to treat the epidemics of CFS, ME and LC that now exist. There is only one person that will get you well and that is you. No-one is better

[†]I read a newspaper article about a merchant bank that decided to target its 100 wealthiest clients for a new investment scheme. A 'round robin' letter was prepared and sent down to the communications department so it could be personalised using the 'mail merge' facility. The minion in that department forgot the substitution; consequently, the 100 wealthiest clients received a letter which opened up 'Dear Rich Bastard'.

motivated. No-one is more in touch with their symptoms and response to interventions than you. No-one knows your body better than you. You must take full responsibility for your own recovery because it is a sad fact that doctors won't. All the Tools of the Trade I give you are freely available (by which I mean you can access them without reference to a doctor), intrinsically safe and of proven effectiveness.

First you must learn to understand *why* you are suffering symptoms and why they are so important and learn to listen to them, not fight them. Do not suppress symptoms with drugs or addictions. Symptoms are the signposts which direct you to the path of recovery. Read on and learn of the mechanisms that result in symptoms because these have obvious implications for treatment. Keep on asking all the right questions because the answers will come, sometimes from the most unlikely direction. I too am constantly asking questions; I too am on a steep learning curve; but I trust and hope this book will launch you to good health.

Take a leap of faith and just do it.

Personal note from Craig

The advice not to fight your symptoms is of the utmost importance, but it does not mean 'surrender' to them. It means work out what they mean and then box clever. We have all been indoctrinated in the Western World that 'fighting an illness' means a particular thing – getting up again and again and pushing through the symptoms of pain and fatigue or whatever. This will not work with CFS, ME and LC. It will only serve to knock you back and often further down. You need to understand and address the mechanisms of those symptoms, and this is what this book is all about. I am reminded of what Napoleon said of Wellington after the Battle of Waterloo (perhaps apocryphally): 'He won by sitting on his arse!' Now I am not suggesting you sit on your arse, because you need to do things, some quite difficult things, in order to get better, but I hope you understand the point. Do not charge headlong into battle against CFS, ME or LC. You will lose. Instead, follow the strategy in this book and fight smart rather than hard.

Chapter 1

The road map* for recovery

We have symptoms for very good reasons – they protect us from ourselves. Without the symptom of pain from a broken leg, we would continue to walk until the bone broke through the skin, infection would set in, and we would die. Symptoms point to underlying pathology, which is why symptom-suppressing prescription drugs are so dangerous. We use addictions to deal with fatigue and stress: caffeine, sugar and cocaine for a short-term hit of false energy; alcohol, nicotine and cannabis to mask symptoms of stress. Any such regular use, points to the start of pathology.

Doctors routinely muddle clinical pictures and diagnoses. A clinical picture is simply a collection of symptoms, but so often these are presented as a diagnosis. Patients tell me they have been 'diagnosed' with irritable bowel syndrome and given symptom-supressing drugs, but the actual diagnosis of food allergy or upper fermenting gut has not been considered. Patients are left with a lifetime of pills, which drive other diseases, instead of being cured by simple dietary changes.

***Historical note:** The Romans knew the value of a good road map. The *Dura-Europos* map is the oldest known map of (a part of) Europe in its original form. It is a fragment of a map drawn onto a leather portion of a shield by a Roman soldier in c 235 AD. It depicts several towns along the northwest coast of the Black Sea. Better still, the *Tabula Peutingeriana*, dating to about 350 AD, plots the extent of the *Cursus publicus*, the Roman road network that ran from Europe and North Africa to West Asia. It is not to scale, or even correct in its orientation – the Mediterranean Sea is a thin sliver and the Italian Peninsula runs east-west – but it did the job, much as the London Underground map does the job today, being itself not to scale nor perfectly oriented. But, the trophy for *the* oldest known road map goes to the Ancient Egyptians: the *Turin Papyrus Map* was drawn around 1160 BC and depicts routes (roads) along dry river beds through a mining region of Thebes.

'Chronic fatigue syndrome' (CFS) is not a diagnosis. It is a clinical picture which results from poor energy delivery mechanisms.

'Myalgic encephalitis' (or 'encephalomyelitis' – ME) is not a diagnosis. It is a clinical picture which results from CFS *and* inflammation. Inflammation occurs when the immune system is activated. This may be for reasons of allergy, autoimmunity, chronic infection, toxicity or healing and repair.

Long Covid (LC) is not a diagnosis. It is the clinical picture of ME but is given the name LC because it follows an acute Covid infection or mRNA gene therapy 'vaccine'.

Fatigue is the symptom that protects us from ourselves

We all have a bucket of energy to spend in a day. If we spend more energy than is in the bucket, then we die.[†]

Spending energy is fun. It gets things done. So, symptoms of fatigue have to be very nasty, or we would push on through. Such symptoms prevent athletes from winning gold medals – they are very effective at saving our lives! This is why 'graded exercise' for CFS and ME is such a nonsense and also dangerous – it kicks another hole in an already small energy bucket. And this is also why pacing (see Chapter 9) is so important – it allows us to spend energy wisely.

At last, after much campaigning, the UK's NICE (National Institute for Health and Care Excellence) has recognised the utter futility and danger of graded exercise therapy (GET) for CFS and ME patients in its new Guideline[1] in which it states that:

> *1.11.14 Do not offer people with ME/CFS:*
> *any programme .... that uses fixed incremental increases in physical activity or exercise, for example, graded exercise therapy.*

[†]**Historical note:** The first recorded example of this is the athlete Pheidippides running from Marathon to Athens after the battle, to announce the Greek victory with the word 'Nenikēkamen!' (Attic: *νενικήκαμεν*; We've won!), whereupon he promptly died of exhaustion.

Before I met him, Craig was persuaded to 'have a go at GET' (as his GP suggested). In typical fashion, he engaged fully and consequently, after 10 months of pushing and falling and pushing again, and falling again, he landed in bed… for nearly five years. Prior to engaging with GET, Craig was perfectly ambulant, and was looking for part-time employment. He could mow his lawn (and his lawn is 80 yards/metres long and at least 4 yards/metres wide) and he could drive his car for, say 3 hours, perfectly safely. He played his beloved tennis with his daughter and son.[‡] All these things, and much more, and many future possibilities, were taken away from him by GET.

Evidence of harm caused by GET was submitted as part of the NICE review of ME/CFS guidance.[2] It concluded that: 'Fifty-one per cent of survey respondents (range 28-82%, n=4338, 8 surveys) reported that GET worsened their health.' Indeed, in one of the those eight related studies ('surveys') reviewed, an astonishing 82% of patients reported a worsening of health following GET.[3] In this paper, authors Keith Geraghty and colleagues, concluded that: '…graded exercise therapy brings about large negative responses in patients (54%–74%).' But I digress. There is more on this in Chapter 23.

Inflammation produces symptoms which protect us from ourselves

Local inflammation is characterised by redness, heat, swelling, pain and loss of function. This makes us spare or rest the afflicted area, so we limp, hold ourselves in an awkward position, find other ways of doing things… or whatever.

General inflammation is characterised by malaise (feeling 'flu like), fever and 'illness behaviour', otherwise known as 'man 'flu'. This makes us want to go to bed, wrap up warm, feel depressed and be antisocial.

[‡]The saying goes, you should leave Oxford with a First, a Blue or a spouse. Craig missed out on an Oxford Blue in Lawn Tennis – he was first reserve in the University Team but never actually played a rubber as none of his team mates were ever injured or sick. However, as Meatloaf says in his song of the same title 'Two out of three ain't bad' and Craig is happy with his First and even happier with his spouse!

The immune system is greatly demanding of energy and, when busy, this kicks an immunological hole in the energy bucket and that leads to more fatigue.

So, this gives us a road map for recovery:

First, spend energy wisely – This is called pacing. It is very boring but essential in the early days.

THEN improve energy delivery mechanisms.

THEN identify the holes in the energy bucket which may be the immunological hole (see Chapter 19) or the emotional hole (often post-traumatic stress – see Chapter 21).

To illustrate the overall principle, I refer to one of our favourite and most apposite quotations:

> *Annual income twenty pounds, annual expenditure nineteen pounds, nineteen and six, result happiness. Annual income twenty pounds, annual expenditure twenty pounds nought and six, result misery.*
>
> Mr Micawber in *David Copperfield* by Charles Dickens

And so, it is with energy:

When the gap is positive, we have energy.

When the gap narrows, we have misery and fatigue.

When the gap is negative, we die.

In treating CFS, ME or LC, and indeed in postponing death, we have to maximise energy delivery mechanisms and minimise useless or unwanted energy expenditure in order to create a positive gap. However, first we have to recognise the symptoms of the above because these will guide us to the best treatments.

Where do you go from here? The road map

As I have said, CFS is not a diagnosis. It is a clinical picture made up of symptoms which result from poor energy delivery mechanisms. Symptoms are found in Chapter 2 and treatments are found in Chapters 3-9.

Likewise, ME and LC are not diagnoses. They are clinical pictures which result from CFS *plus* inflammation. Inflammation occurs when the immune system is activated. Again as I have said, this may be for reasons of allergy, autoimmunity, chronic infection, toxicity or healing and repair. Symptoms of ME and LC are found in Chapter 10. You must still do all the treatments in Chapters 3-9, and then add in the treatments found in Chapters 11-20 that are relevant to your case.

CFS, ME and LC sufferers must *all* consider the emotional holes in the energy bucket (see Chapter 21). CFS, ME and LC sufferers can expect to get better, as shown in Chapter 22 (the journey to recovery). The politics of CFS, ME and LC are discussed briefly in Chapter 23.

Summary

- To overcome CFS, ME or LC, you need a road map.
- Craig says: Do *not* try random interventions 'willy nilly'[§]. This is from my own experience before I met Sarah.
- This book is a road map developed over decades of experience and academic study.
- This road map works.

[§]**Linguistic note:** 'Willy-nilly' derives from the obsolete phrase 'will I, nill I', or 'I am willing, I am unwilling'.

Chapter 2

Chronic fatigue syndrome

The symptoms of poor energy delivery mechanisms

I am somewhat exhausted; I wonder how a battery feels when it pours electricity into a non-conductor?

Sir Arthur Conan Doyle, British writer and physician (22 May 1859 – 7 July 1930)

Most, if not all, of my CFS, ME and LC patients know exactly how that battery feels. These are the symptoms described in this chapter. It is important to understand these symptoms because the starting point to treat all such is the same – improve energy delivery mechanisms.

Poor energy delivery to the body

Energy is produced in almost every cell in the body.

Poor energy delivery results in physical fatigue. We all feel tired at the end of the day, but pathological fatigue is characterised by delay – overdo it one day and we 'pay' for it the next day, and possibly for several days. This is called 'post-exertional malaise'. Part of the mechanism of this has to do with lactic acid. Over 90% of all our energy comes from aerobic metabolism – we 'burn' fuel, acetate with oxygen in our mitochondrial engines to make energy.* One molecule of acetate creates 32-36 molecules of ATP, the energy molecule, depending on the efficiency of our engines. If our engines are overwhelmed, then we move temporarily to anaerobic energy production. This is horribly inefficient: 1 molecule of acetate fuel generates just 2 molecules of ATP by this route. The anaerobic process also makes lactic acid. Not only is this painful, but it also blocks our mitochondrial engines. This might seem like a rotten piece of design, but actually it protects us from ourselves – this is the mechanism by which we are stopped in our tracks by pain and fatigue before we go into negative energy balance and die!

This mechanism further explains the imperative to pace activity. Lactic acid is painful and has to be converted back to acetate. This process is called the Cori cycle and it takes 6 molecules to achieve. Think of ATP, the energy molecule, as money. To achieve an

*__Footnote:__ There is much more about mitochondria and their function in Chapter 5 but a brief summary is called for here in order to cement understanding of this key biochemical process and its implications for CFS, ME and LC sufferers. Mitochondrial failure is *the* central cause of CFS, ME and LC. The biochemistry, Krebs cycle etcetera alluded to here is one that doctors and chemists learn the night before the examination, and then forget. It is very detailed and one does not need to know those details but rather one needs only to know the overview and the implications of all of this to you, the sufferer.

The dominant role of mitochondria is to produce ATP (adenosine-triphosphate). This is achieved (in normal circumstances) by oxidising (or 'burning') acetate (derived from glucose and fatty acids) in the presence of oxygen. This is known as aerobic respiration. ATP is crucial to all body functions: it is the energy molecule and powers all such body functions. In these (good) normal circumstances, the word equation for this process of aerobic respiration is:

Glucose + Oxygen → Carbon dioxide + Water + 32-36 molecules of ATP (aerobic respiration)

However, when one (anyone) has overdone things, then the system moves temporarily to **an**aerobic (without oxygen) respiration. For CFS, ME and LC sufferers, this switch to anaerobic respiration happens much more quickly than usual (for example, maybe walking five paces will cause such a switch) and also it takes much longer for the CFS, ME and LC sufferer to switch back to aerobic respirations (often days, if not longer). The problem with anaerobic respiration is that it only produces 2 molecules of ATP as seen in its word equation as below:

Glucose → 2 Lactic acid + 2 ATP (anaerobic respiration)

But it is worse than that. As already mentioned, the lactic acid causes pain (the burn that athletes know so well) and also it takes 6 molecules of ATP to convert the lactic acid back to acetate, ready to be oxidised in aerobic respiration. One has effectively lost 4 molecules of ATP in this transaction. So, you are left with pain and a long recovery period from that pain. I have written extensively on this subject and you will find the links to my three published papers at the start of Chapter 5. You do *not* need to know the detail. But perhaps it will reassure you that the detail *is* there. Once you feel better, maybe you could go back and read those three papers and understand why you do feel better.

action we can 'borrow' 2 molecules of ATP, but we have to pay it back with 6 molecules. This is like borrowing energy from a loan shark.

Poor energy delivery to muscles

Poor energy delivery to muscles results in weak muscles with no stamina. Overdo things slightly and you get lactic acid burn. This is painful.

Poor energy delivery to the brain

Many sufferers of CFS, ME and LC are convinced that they are developing dementia. Indeed, dementia is the symptom that occurs when energy delivery to the brain is impaired. It can be reversed by improving energy delivery mechanisms. We all know the symptoms: foggy brain, inability to concentrate or multitask and, sometimes, an inability to find the right word, or maybe use of 'opposite' words to those intended, poor short-term memory and so on. Some individuals cannot even follow the plot of a film on TV. It is scary.

Personal note from Craig

At one point, in around 2001, I was totally bedridden, and this lasted for a number of years. My cognitive ability was so low that at one point I could not count from one to 10. This level of brain fog lasted for about 10 months. It was very scary. I thought my brain was totally shot. It wasn't – but it did need vastly improved energy delivery. And when that energy started to get through, my brain fog lifted, and I began to help Sarah with her website and her books. During the first Covid lockdown, I wrote a mathematics book, *Rockets and Raindrops*, about varying mass problems. This was one of my lifetime ambitions and for two brief periods, *Rockets and Raindrops* was seventh and 15th in Amazon worldwide sales in the 'Applied Mathematics' category, due to large orders from Japanese schools! My point is that I truly believe that, no matter how bad things are, you can always improve. You can still realise dreams. I was desolate during the early 2000s and had given up on any kind of recovery. If someone had predicted all of the above, I would have probably sworn at them and thrown whatever I could at them. But I stuck with the road map, as provided by Sarah, and I was supported and loved by my incredible wife, Penny, and spurred on by my amazing children, Gina and Conor, who 'took' me for who I was, as children do. Please, dear reader, never ever give up. There are good days ahead of you, waiting for you to be there. By the way, as of today (13 November 2023), *Rockets and Raindrops* is placed at position 5105 in the 'Applied Mathematics' category on Amazon.

Low brain energy can also result in intolerance of light, noise, smell and sometimes touch. The business of processing information requires large amounts of energy. About one third of the resources of the brain go into transforming the signal that arises from light on the retina to a three-dimensional depiction of the world around us. My worst afflicted patients only feel comfortable in a darkened room.

Then the brain gives us symptoms to stop us spending energy, such as depression (which makes us antisocial) and procrastination.

I think the symptom of feeling stressed is one that the brain gives us when it knows it does not have the energy to deal with demands.

Poor energy delivery to the heart

Poor energy delivery to the heart manifests in two ways – with POTs (postural orthostatic tachycardia syndrome) and pain. Heart muscle pain is called angina.

POTs

The heart is a muscle – impair energy delivery and it can no longer beat powerfully. This presents with low blood pressure. I reckon a BP of 100/60 mm Hg or less is pathological.

There is much less work involved in pumping blood round the body on the flat, so the severely afflicted person spends their life horizontal. We all know this. We rest sitting down with our feet up. Problems arise when we stand up (the 'postural orthostatic' bit) – circulating blood in the vertical position means the heart has to increase output by about 20%. However, our sick CFS heart cannot increase energy delivery mechanisms – it is already working to its full ability. The only way it can increase cardiac output in the short term is to beat faster (the 'tachycardia' bit). But beating faster is also demanding of energy; this is not sustainable. It beats less strongly, blood pressure falls and, unless our sick patient lies down quickly, they faint and drop unconscious. This mechanism has been confirmed by Dr Peckerman who measured cardiac output by impedance cardiography and found that:

> *...cardiac output in healthy people will vary from 7 litres per min when lying down to 5 litres per min when standing. In healthy people this drop is not enough to affect function. But in CFSs the drop may be from 5 litres lying down to 3.5 litres standing up. At this level the sufferer has a cardiac output which causes borderline organ failure. In CFS the low cardiac output is caused by poor muscle function and therefore strictly speaking is a cardiomyopathy. This means the function of the heart will be very abnormal, but traditional tests of heart failure, such as ECG, ECHOs, angiograms etc, will be normal.*[1]

I have a few patients for whom the symptoms of POTs do not resolve despite doing all they can to improve energy delivery mechanisms. It may be due to an infection of the vagus nerve; this is impossible to prove but biologically plausible since herpes viruses target nerves. Indeed, Michael Van Elzakker has hypothesised that in ME, which is driven by infection (that is to say, the clinical picture is one of poor energy delivery *and* inflammation), the vagus nerve has been infected and this *also* results in POTs.[2]

Another possibility is that this autonomic dysfunction may be related to over-breathing (see Chapter 6: Oxygen).

Some of these patients respond to TENS stimulation of the vagus nerve. This is work in progress.

Angina

The term 'angina' simply means pain in the heart. It is caused by lactic acid burn. The cardiologists recognise the clinical picture of angina as a result of poor blood supply to the heart when demands exceed oxygen delivery. There is a switch into metabolism without oxygen (anaerobic) and lactic acid is painful.

The patient with atherosclerosis (blocked arteries) immediately feels the pain, stops activity, and the oxygen supply is restored as demand falls and a normal mitochondrial aerobic engine clears the lactic acid. This take seconds to minutes. It is a very different picture for the mitochondriac – that is, the CFS sufferer. They get lactic acid burn when energy demand exceeds energy delivery because the mitochondrial engine is slow – too slow even to clear the lactic acid. They suffer angina which lasts minutes to hours. They are not diagnosed with angina by cardiologists because the clinical picture does not fit and imaging of the arteries (angiography) shows coronary arteries to be normal. They are instead diagnosed (please try not to laugh at this point) with 'atypical chest pain'. But we now know this is loan-shark pain – not a diagnosis, but a clinical picture.

Poor energy delivery to the liver

At rest the brain consumes 20% of total body energy production, the heart 7% and the liver up to 27%. Much of this is to maintain our internal homeostasis (metabolic balance), including detoxification – that is, the clearing out of unusable/toxic substances that we take in and our body creates. Poor energy delivery means we become slow detoxifiers and symptomatic of this is intolerance of drugs, including alcohol, antidepressants, statins and many more. Many patients are told that their symptoms can be improved with antidepressants, they then find they are intolerant of these, stop them and are accused of not complying with treatment. Further medical support may then be withheld.

Poor energy delivery to the immune system

Our immune system is our standing army with which we fight acute infection. Armies need white cell officers and soldiers with mobility, intelligence, communication skills, weapons and firepower. Having destroyed the enemy, our white cell troops then heal and repair the damage. These processes all require energy. Poor energy delivery is a cause of immune suppression. It may also lead to poor decision making, risking civil war (autoimmunity) or damage to non-threatening tourists (allergy).

Poor energy delivery to cells and organs

If energy delivery to cells is slow, then organs go slow. Ultimately this leads to organ failure, degeneration and cancer.

Summary

All the consequences of poor energy delivery described in this chapter explain why improving energy delivery is the starting point for treating not just fatigue syndromes but all disease processes. In summary:

- Poor energy delivery affects all parts of the body and gives rise to symptoms.
- These symptoms include:
  - pain
  - fatigue
  - weakness
  - brain fog
  - angina
  - POTs
  - poor detoxification and subsequent lack of tolerance of drugs
  - weakened immune system and
  - (in the longer term) organ failure leading to degeneration and cancer.

So, having described what poor energy delivery can look like, let's go on to describe the mechanisms of such poor energy delivery and how to fix them. We must understand the mechanisms in order to put them right.

Chapter 3

The mechanisms of poor energy delivery and how to treat them

This chapter gives an overview.* Don't expect to understand all of this now. Reading the rest of the book will make it all clear, but it is useful at the outset to see what goes wrong and how to fix it, in general terms, before we delve into more detail. You may find Table 3.1, which summaries this overview, the most perused section of this book in time.

I like to use the car analogy. For our car to go well we need: Fuel in the tank, a functioning engine, an accelerator pedal, a gear box, service and repair, and regular use. The equivalents in our body are: What we eat and drink, the metabolic systems and

***Note from Craig:** In liking overviews, Sarah is in good company. René Descartes (French philosopher, scientist and mathematician, 31 March 1596 – 11 February 1650), said of Pierre de Fermat (French mathematician, between 31 October and 6 December 1607 – 12 January 1665): 'It cannot be denied that he has had many exceptional ideas, and that he is a highly intelligent man. For my part, however, I have always been taught to take a broad overview of things, in order to be able to deduce from them general rules, which might be applicable elsewhere.' Pierre de Fermat is perhaps most famous now for his 'Last Theorem' which he described in a note, without proof, in the margin of a copy of Diophantus's *Arithmetica*. After 358 years of effort by mathematicians, the first successful proof of said Last Theorem was released in 1994 by Andrew Wiles (English Mathematician, 11 April 1953 –) and formally published in 1995. However, Fermat did so much more than write down his Last Theorem without proof. One does not have Sir Isaac Newton (English mathematician, physicist, astronomer, alchemist, theologian and author, 25 December 1642 – 20 March 1726/27) say that his ideas about calculus came directly from 'Fermat's way of drawing tangents' if one is not a truly remarkable mathematician, as Fermat was.

Note from Sarah: Can you tell, dear reader, that Craig has moved on from an inability to count from one to 10. I have to stop him these days!

processes that turn fuel into energy, an optimally functioning thyroid gland and adrenal glands, sufficient sleep and detoxification processes, and appropriately paced exercise. Table 3.1 provides the detail together with how to fix the problems that arise.

Table 3.1: Overview of energy delivery and how to fix the problems that occur in CFS/ME/LC

Car	Your body	How to fix this
Fuel in the tank	The fuel must be primarily ketones	PK diet (see Chapter 4)
	An upper gut that can digest and absorb	Sort out the upper fermenting gut (see Chapter 4 for what this is) with the PK diet plus: Vitamin C 5 grams (g) during the day Lugol's iodine 15 % 3 drops at night NB: Vitamin C and iodine must be separated by at least 2 hours as they knock each other out
	A basic package of supplements to compensate for the deficiencies of modern food (Appendices)	You need a non-fermenting upper gut to absorb these: Multivitamins Minerals Essential fatty acids (omega-6 and omega-3) Vitamin D 10,000 iu
The engine	The mitochondria engines (see Chapter 5) must work and to do this they need the right fuel in the tank – primarily ketones. Yes, this is repetition, but this is often the single most important intervention!	PK diet
	Good oxygen delivery to mitochondria	Correct your breathing by always breathing through your nose, learn diaphragmatic breathing, slow your breathing so you have a controlled pause of 30, ideally 40, seconds; this improves oxygen delivery to the tissues (see Chapter 6)

Table 3.1: *Cont'd*

Car	Your body	How to fix this
Spark plugs	The raw materials to function	Magnesium 300 mg (with breakfast) Vitamin D 10,000 iu for its absorption (with breakfast)
Oil	Co-enzyme Q 10 and niacinamide (vitamin B3)	Co-enzyme Q10 100 mg (with breakfast) Niacinamide 1500 mg (with breakfast)
Fuel delivery	Fuel delivery into mitochondria, which are within cells	Acetyl L carnitine 1 g (with breakfast)
		D-ribose 5-15 g daily – this is the raw material to make de novo ATP should one really over-do things; it helps prevent post-exertional malaise. NB: One can use this as a rescue remedy – Craig carries 5 g dissolved in mineral water in a hip flask, just in case
	Freedom from blocking by: a) lactic acid	Must pace activity – yes, I know this is boring!
	b) toxins from the upper fermenting gut (alcohol, D lactate, hydrogen sulphide, ammoniacal compounds)	Sort out the upper fermenting gut with: PK diet Vitamin C 5 g by day Lugol's iodine 15% 3 drops at night
	c) malondialdehyde† and other such from poor antioxidant status	Make sure you use ketones as a fuel (sugar as a fuel generates free radicals) – PK diet again. Addition antioxidant glutathione 250 mg
	d) social drugs: sugar, alcohol, caffeine, nicotine, chocolate as well as street drugs	Addictions are good servants but bad masters. Use very occasionally to enhance a jolly
	e) prescription drugs: the vast majority do not address root causes and accelerate underlying pathology	Work out if/why you need these. See our book *Ecological Medicine* for guidance on this. With its help, get symptom free and aim to stop them all

†**Footnote to table:** Malondialdehyde (MDA) is one of the final products of polyunsaturated fatty acids peroxidation in the cells. This showed up very commonly in the tests as done by Dr John Maclaren Howard of translocator function (see page 55). This test is currently available from the Academy of Nutritional Medicine (http://aonm.org/mitochondrial-testing/) and there are other tests of poor antioxidant status that can be useful, such as the Genova tests of oxidative stress markers.

Table 3.1: *Cont'd*

Car	Your body	How to fix this
	f) pesticides and volatile organic compounds	Avoid Get rid of stored toxins with heating regimes – Epsom salt baths, infrared sauna-ing, keeping warm, sunshine, heat belts or lamps – then wash off (see Chapter 14: Detoxing)
	g) toxic metals	Avoid Measure Get rid of stored metals with chelation and food clays (see Chapter 14)
	Improve ability to detox	Glutathione 250 mg Vitamin B12 injections (great for the foggy brain) Sulphur as DMSO (dimethylsulphoxide) Methylation – measure homocysteine
	Avoid electromagnetic radiation: 5G, mobile phones, cordless phones and wifi – disrupts the electrical potential across all cell membranes	Avoid See my webpage for how[1]
	Reduce inflammation – it increases the friction in the system and blocks mitochondria with inflammatory mediators	Reduce inflammation as shown in Chapter 13
	Get all the above in the correct 3D position – this requires fourth phase water (see page 155)	Heat from infrared (keeping warm, sunshine, heat belts or lamps) DMSO 20 ml daily
	Re-educate the mitochondria	Micro-immunotherapy remedies MISEN and MIREG (see Chapter 19)
The accelerator pedal	Thyroid gland: The underactive thyroid is common and thyroid hormones work by stimulating mitochondria so you must sort these out first	Thyroid glandulars (see Chapter 7)

Table 3.1: *Cont'd*

Car	Your body	How to fix this
The gear box	Adrenal glands: Adrenal fatigue is common	Adrenal glandulars (see Chapter 7): Pregnenolone 25-100 mg DHEA 25-100 mg Ashwaganda 1-4 g Ginseng 1-4 g
Servicing and repair	Sleep: Aim for at least 8, preferably 9, hours' sleep during the hours of darkness, more in winter	See Chapter 8
	Tool box – the methylation cycle	Measure homocysteine – should lie between 5 and 10 mcmol/l NB: Everyone should know their homocysteine
Use it or lose it	Exercise and pacing – we lose muscle with age and disease	Do the right sort of exercise to build up and/or slow down muscle loss (see Chapter 9)

What to do first: Fixing problems in the right order

Not only are all the steps in Table 3.1 essential for recovery but they must also all be done in the right order. You cannot correct mitochondrial function without *both* the right fuel in the tank (the PK diet) *and* an upper gut which can absorb the necessary raw materials (so, sort out the upper fermenting gut). The PK diet must therefore be done *before* the mitochondrial support package.

In addition, you cannot correct thyroid and adrenal function until you have mitochondria in a fit state to respond. So, the mitochondria must be corrected before you move onto the thyroid and adrenals.

This all takes time. Furthermore, any one of the above interventions may trigger a 'healing crisis', where you feel worse before you feel better (see Appendix 2).

With *all* of the above, start low and build up slow. The sicker you are the lower you start and the slower you go.

You may get worse initially. I call these 'DDD (diet, detox and die-off) reactions' – see Appendix 2. The sickest patients are the most likely to experience such reactions. Sadly they must expect the bumpiest ride. This is when symptoms which should signpost recovery make life very confusing and you need to be convinced of the correctness of your interventions to stay on the wagon.

Table 3.2: An approximate time scale

The starting point	What	Timing
Endurance athletes who wish to improve their performance	PK diet and get keto-adapted (Chapter 4)	1-2 weeks, carry on for life
	Then take vitamin C and iodine to sort the upper fermenting gut	1 week, carry on for life
	Then start the Basic Package of supplements (page 43)	Carry on for life Rehydrate with Sunshine salt after exercise
Younger athletes	Young athletes do not have mitochondrial problems – training stimulates more mitochondria i.e. a bigger engine; this is reflected by bigger muscles	Rehydrate with Sunshine salt after exercise
Vegetarians and vegans	Ditto above *but* the raw materials for mitochondria we get from eating other mitochondria, and these are rich in meat, fish and eggs	Mitochondrial supplements (page 60) are a good idea Carry on for life
	Stay fit with the right sort of exercise	For life (Chapter 9)

Table 3.2: *Cont'd*

The starting point	What	Timing
Ageing old crones like me… as energy declines	As per athletes *but* mitochondria also determine the ageing process	Address mitochondrial issues as above and carry on with Groundhog Basic (Appendix 1) for life
	Sleep – if quality diminishes take melatonin	3-9 mg melatonin at night Carry on for life
	Adrenal fatigue is very common over the age of 60 – take pregnenolone (dubbed the memory hormone)	50 mg pregnenolone (with breakfast) Take for as long as needed to ensure 8-9 hours of good quality sleep between the hours of 10 pm and 7 am
	The underactive thyroid is common, especially in women at the menopause – take thyroid glandulars	Takes 2-3 months to correct – once you have the 'sweet spot' carry on for life (see Chapter 7)
	Stay fit with the right sort of exercise. As you grow older you can stay fit and well but you have to be disciplined and work harder to achieve such	For life (Chapter 9)
Functioning at 70/100 on the Bell disability scale (see Appendix 5)	All the above At this level you may be able to hold down a sedentary job but you have to spend weekends and holidays resting	Should be able to bring in all the above interventions over a few weeks to months
Functioning at 50/100 on the Bell disability scale (see Appendix 5)	All the above – but expect nasty DDD reactions (Appendix 2)	PK diet and sort the upper fermenting gut over 1 month Mitochondrial regimes – 2 months Thyroid and adrenals – 3 months
Functioning at 30/100 on the Bell disability scale (see Appendix 5)	Ditto When this ill it is much more likely that there are inflammatory issues as well and serious toxicity issues. You will not be able to hold down a job and you will need financial benefits (see Appendix 6)	Ditto above Should there be a DDD reaction (Appendix 2) then do all the above but even more slowly. There is a particularly difficult balancing act where there is an underactive thyroid with ketogenic hypoglycaemia – see Chapter 7

The starting point	What	Timing
Functioning at 20/100 on the Bell disability scale (see Appendix 5)	Ditto Very difficult At this level of illness you do not have the energy to look after yourself let alone put in place all the necessary regimes for recovery. You need money, care and carers. And all of these may be very difficult to come by, but I know no other path to tread. You have to be a very patient patient. However, all the above prevent cancer, heart disease and dementia – so you can look forward to better times ahead!	Ditto above Expect DDD reactions (Appendix 2) Go slow

Summary

- The mechanisms of poor energy delivery include:
  - The wrong diet
  - Poorly functioning mitochondria
  - Poor oxygen delivery at the tissue level
  - Poor thyroid and adrenal function
  - Not enough good quality sleep
  - Not enough of the right sort of exercise.
- These mechanisms can be fixed by:
  - The PK diet
  - Pacing
  - Breathing exercises
  - Various supplements to support mitochondrial, thyroid and adrenal function
  - Avoiding addictions, prescription drugs, toxic metals and pesticides and other toxins
  - Improving detoxification and methylation
  - Reducing inflammation
  - Doing the right sort of exercise, when you are able, and only when this is sustainable.

Chapter 4

First steps

The paleo-ketogenic (PK) diet, sorting the upper fermenting gut, and the Basic Package of supplements

The three steps to undertake first, in the correct order as explained in this chapter, are:

1. The PK diet – get into ketosis and balance up total calories needed with protein and carbs.
2. Sort out the upper fermenting gut with the PK diet, vitamin C and fasting.
3. Start the Basic Package of supplements, to be taken for life.

WHAT TO EAT AND WHEN

The Cure is in the Kitchen.

Dr Sherry Rogers, environmental physician

The paleo-ketogenic (PK) diet is non-negotiable, as I will explain. I spend more time talking about diet and cooking than all other subjects put together. Changing one's diet is the first thing one must do and the most difficult. It is also the most important thing to do for good health. In fact, the very derivation of the word 'diet' gives us a clue as to just how important it is. It is of Greek origin: *diaita*, originally 'way of life or regimen' related to *diaitasthai* meaning 'lead one's life'. As you will learn, 'doing' the PK diet is a change to how one leads one's life.

Why the PK diet is non-negotiable

The following is a very brief overview, which you can skip over if you simply want the 'How' of the PK diet. For readers who want to know more, there is much more detail in our book *Paleo-Ketogenic: The Why and the How* but I give the basics of 'What' and 'Why' here. Please follow this guidance – it is born out of bitter experience.

So very briefly, to give you the 'What', a paleo-ketogenic diet follows paleo principles in avoiding the food products of civilisation – principally dairy and grains plus anything processed – and ketogenic principles in largely avoiding sugar and starchy carbohydrates. You can eat some of these foods so long as you are in ketosis most of the time. 'Ketogenic' describes this diet because fuelling our bodies with fat and fibre generates 'ketones' to fuel our bodies and puts us into 'ketosis', the healthy metabolic state in which our body is burning fuel from fat and fibre, not carbs/glucose. Please see the box below for the benefits of ketosis.

Research showing the benefits of ketosis

If you need to convince yourself, or others, of the benefits of the PK diet, then please see the medical research page of the website 'Ketogenic Diet Resource' (www.ketogenic-diet-resource.com/medical-research.html). This page lists dozens of studies showing benefits for the following conditions:

- Alzheimer's disease
- Autism
- Bipolar disorder
- Cancer
- Diabetes, type 1
- Diabetes, type 2
- Epilepsy
- Fatty liver disease
- GERD/Reflux/Heartburn
- Heart disease

- Insulin resistance/Metabolic syndrome
- Migraine headaches
- Multiple sclerosis
- Parkinson's disease
- Schizophrenia/Schizoaffective disorder
- Weight loss.

The PK diet is *not* a high-protein diet as I will explain later in this chapter when I talk about how to calculate your individual protein needs.

Then, to give you a very brief overview of the 'Why', humans evolved over 2.5 million years eating a paleo-ketogenic diet. This is the diet best suited to our bowels, bodies and brains. If we wish to live to our full potential in terms of quality and quantity of life, this is the diet naturally selected by survival of the fittest. We humans can live on two fuels – fats and carbohydrates – and this has given us great adaptability. Indeed, we can live on a greater variety of foods than almost any other mammal. However, fuelling our bodies with a high-carbohydrate diet leads to the fundamental problems fuelling chronic disease today:

- Carbohydrates are addictive.
- Excess carbohydrates cause metabolic syndrome leading to insulin resistance, pre-diabetes and type 2 diabetes.
- A high-carb diet overwhelms the stomach's ability to digest, leading to the upper fermenting gut (UFG) – see below.
- A high-carb diet overwhelms the liver, leading to a hormone response – principally chronically high insulin (hyperinsulinaemia) – that inhibits the burning of fat.
- It also means our 'glycogen sponge' – the limited sugar storage space in our muscles and liver – is constantly saturated so too much sugar constantly spills into our bloodstream where it sticks to arteries, feeds cancer cells and infections, and drives dementia and degenerative disease.

Remember, outside autumn primitive humans had no choice but to eat a paleo-ketogenic diet and this would have been largely comprised of raw meat and/or raw fish and shellfish, depending on where these early humans lived. That was it. You may think this a boring diet, but boredom is a word that means people are missing their carb addiction!

> *My job is to get you well, not to entertain you.*
>
> Yours Truly
>
> (Some say that quoting oneself lacks humility. It is a good job then that Craig included the above!)

The carnivore diet

For some of the sickest patients, especially those in whom allergy is suspected, we have to return to a very primitive carnivore diet to allow them to recover. This is because no plant wants to be eaten so all contain substances that are toxic. In essence, the primitive carnivore diet is as below (see *Paleo-Ketogenic: The Why and the How* for more detail).

Drinks:

- Water, flat or fizzy
- Black tea and coffee (away from mealtimes)
- Bone broth – with a pinch of Sunshine salt (see below)

Meals:

- At first you should eat meat only
- If you are sure you are not allergic to fish, then add it in
- If you are sure you are not allergic to eggs, then add them in too.

The PK diet: The How

Back to the PK diet. An essential part of the 'How' of this diet is to access bone marrow. Perhaps this is what drove primitive man to using tools to smash open this treasure chest of fat and micronutrients and so the clever ones survived? Neanderthal man had a larger brain than modern man.

As my patients often hear in the consulting room: 'Guess what? I am not going to live my life eating raw meat and raw fish just so that I can live to a great age.' We all have to work out a compromise diet that gets the best of both the paleo and modern worlds. And that is going to be different for everyone and will change with age. For me, greed gets in the way – I love good food. So, we all need a starting point which can then be relaxed or tightened up depending on our age and health/disease state. Younger, healthy, physically active people can take more liberties than old, sick ones. I find myself in the old, healthy category and so I am still no paragon of virtue.

What to eat

A reasonable starting point for most is the following.

You can eat as much as you like of:

- Fats – Saturated fats for energy, such as lard, butter or ideally ghee (so long as you are sure you are not allergic to dairy – I am … dammit), goose fat, coconut oil, palm oil.
- Oils – Unsaturated fats which are also fuels but contain essential omega-3, omega-6 and omega-9 fatty acids. Hemp oil is ideal, containing the perfect proportion of omega-6 to omega-3 – that is, 4:1. These oils must be cold pressed and not used for cooking or you risk 'flipping' them into toxic trans fats. Only cook with biochemically stable, saturated fats. (See *Paleo-Ketogenic: The Why and the How* for more on good and bad fats.) I use vegan block as a butter substitute.
- Fibre – This is often included in the carb count of foods and leads to some confusion. Eat enough fibre to ensure that when you are crapping you do so twice daily to produce a turd effortlessly (no straining), cucumber-size, no cracks, no balling, soft and inoffensive. To be precise, type 4 on the Bristol stool chart[1] – and yes, you can purchase the T-shirt so emblazoned with the Bristol stool chart. Denis Burkitt, consultant surgeon, studied African societies and observed that indigenous Africans eating their traditional diet did not suffer from Western diseases and, indeed, these peoples did squat twice daily and produce said turds. He wrote a book, *Don't Forget Fibre in your Diet*, which became an international bestseller.[2] To achieve that which colorectal surgeons dream of you need to consume a quarter of a PK loaf daily (again, see *Paleo-Ketogenic – The Why and the How* plus below) or its fibre

equivalent. Then invest in a squatty potty – I was delighted to read that some have 'motion-sensitive lights'. A high-fibre diet means that fermentation of such in the large bowel generates vitamin K.
- Foods that are less than 5% carbohydrate – The most important are:
    - Linseed – This makes great bread and is also an excellent base for muesli and porridge being high in fibre (see our book *Paleo-Ketogenic: The Why and the How*).
    - Coconut cream – Grace coconut milk is head and shoulders above all others with a 2% carb content. It is a great alternative to dairy. It is available from Amazon and I stock it in my Online Sales Website (see Useful resources, page 303).
    - Brazil and pecan nuts.
    - Salad (lettuce, cucumber, tomato, pepper etc); avocado pear and olives (phew! I love them both).
    - Green leafy vegetables.
    - Mushrooms and fungi – A difficulty with this diet is eating enough fat. These foods are great for frying as they mop up delicious, saturated fats. (I fry mushrooms in my beef dripping every morning with my bacon and eggs – Craig.)
    - Fermented foods such as sauerkraut and kefir, since the carb content has been fermented out by microbes.

Please note again, this is *not* a high-protein diet. While advocating meat, fish, shellfish and eggs, we should not consume too much as excessive amounts can be converted back to carbohydrate. Essentially, too much protein can be converted into sugars via a process called gluconeogenesis. I explain later in this chapter (page 35) how to calculate your personal daily needs though our bodies are good at knowing intuitively what our needs are once we have dealt with any addictions. (If you want more detail on this, again refer to *Paleo-Ketogenic: The Why and the How*.)

Other points to note are:
- Salt – You need 1 tsp (5 grams (g)) daily. A PK diet demands more added salt than Western diets since there is so much salt hidden in processed food. Ideally, use Sunshine salt. I have put this together so that it contains all essential minerals from sodium and selenium to magnesium and manganese, together with 5,000 iu vitamin D and 5 mg vitamin B12 in a 5-g (1 tsp) dose. (See Useful resources, page 305.)

- Coffee and tea in moderation.
- **Avoid foods of 10% or more carbohydrate** as they switch on addictive eating. I know. I too am an addict. This includes all grains, pulses, fruits and their juices, and many nuts and seeds. In particular, avoid all junk food which is characterised by its high-carb content and addictive potential, including crisps (sorry Craig[*]).

Also avoid:
- all sweeteners, natural or artificial, because these simply switch on physical and psychological craving for sugar.
- all dairy products, apart from butter or ghee if you are not allergic.
- all gluten grains.

Both dairy and gluten grains are common allergens and this drives inflammation.

Testing for ketosis

Ketosis is the metabolic state where the majority of the body's energy supply comes in the form of ketone bodies, derived from fat and fibre. This is in contrast with a state of 'glycolysis' where blood glucose provides the majority of the energy supply. Ketosis has many benefits (see Box) including improving energy levels because mitochondria run more efficiently on ketones – the heart and brain run up to 25% more efficiently burning ketones compared with sugar.

Make sure you are in ketosis through testing. As explained, ketones arise through our bodies burning fat. This generates three types of ketone that can be measured in different ways:
- Beta hydroxybutyric acid: This is present in, and can be measured in, the blood; this

[*]**Explanatory note:** Before becoming 'PK-adapted', crisps were my addiction. I ate at least six normal-sized bags of ready-salted crisps each and every day. (See how, even now, I try to rationalise this addiction by the use of the phrase 'normal-sized' as though I am saying to my inner self 'It wasn't that bad, Craig!'). I even had a stash of 12 bags in my wardrobe, 'just in case'! I gave up crisps overnight. One Monday, I threw away all 'my' crisps, stashed in various rooms of our house, and I have not eaten even a single crisp since then. I know that eating even one packet of crisps will trigger the addiction and so I simply never eat them.

is the most accurate measure of ketosis, but testing strips are expensive. I am mean and a wimp, so I do not use this method.
- Acetoacetate: This is excreted in the urine. Testing is cheap and easy with urine keto-stix but, as the body becomes more efficient at matching ketone production to demand, urine tests may show false negatives.
- Acetone: This is exhaled and can be measured with breath testing. This is my preferred method as you can easily test after every meal to ensure you have not overdone the carbs (see Useful Resources on page 303 for details of ketone breath meters).

Trouble-shooting the ketone breath test

If your diet is sufficiently low in carbs, expect to blow 2-4 parts per million (ppm) of ketones. However, the body will always use sugar in preference to ketones. This means that *any* amount of ketones in the breath indicates that you are in ketosis.

If you blow very high levels of ketones – e.g. up to 10 ppm – this is not harmful. It may be for one or more of these reasons:
- When stressed, there is an outpouring of adrenalin and this stimulates fat burning.
- Over-dosing with thyroid hormones may cause high levels of ketones.
- Fasting: Even on a PK diet you consume some carbohydrates. All plants contain some carbs. With fasting you get *all* your calories from fat, so ketones are higher. This illustrates the point that even in mild ketosis you will be using some sugars as a fuel – that is fine. Glycogen in meat is negligible.
- Contamination as listed below.

You can get false positive results for any of these possible reasons:
- If you have consumed any alcohol in the previous 24 hours (depending on how much!): The mechanism used to measure ketones is the same as that for measuring alcohol.
- If you have an upper fermenting gut (see page 40), as this too produces alcohol.
- If you use a product containing alcohol: Any products containing alcohol may give a positive result. I checked this myself with an alcohol wipe (often used for hand

sanitising) to clean the mouthpiece and this gave a high reading.

- If there is contamination from volatile organic compounds (VOCs): The meter measure parts per million (ppm), meaning it is very sensitive. You only need a tiny amount of contaminant to upset the result. Many household cleaners contain VOCs which may register on the meter.

You can also get false negative results.

- If you have had anything to eat or drink in the preceding 20 minutes, then that may affect the test. For example, I know if I have a sip of coffee then that may be followed by a negative reading.

Then you need to be aware:

- The actual figure may not reflect blood levels of ketones. This is partly because blood ketones are different (beta hydroxy butyric acid, as described above) whereas breath ketones are acetones.
- The result may not square with urine ketones. Again, this is because urine ketones are different (acetoacetate). It is common to see ketones on a breath test, but the urine test be negative. Also, with time, the body gets better at matching energy demands to delivery, so fewer ketones are 'wasted' through urinary losses.

Understanding ketosis

Being in ketosis is *not* dangerous. Most doctors do not know or understand physiological ketosis. They only know about diabetic ketoacidosis and may panic if you tell them you are in ketosis.

Ketosis is *only* a medical problem if you are diabetic and your blood sugars are running high (either because your medication is insufficient or because you are consuming too many carbs). For example, a blood sugar above 10 mmol/l and/or the presence of sugar in your urine *IS* a medical emergency.

Bear in mind that the DIY home tests for blood sugar rely on a test that employs glucose oxidase. Vitamin C cross-reacts, so if you are taking vitamin C to bowel tolerance (see section at the end of this chapter, page 44) your blood will be saturated with vitamin C and this may give false highs. My experience is that this may be 2-3 mmol/l higher than the actual blood glucose – that is to say, an apparent reading of 7-8 mmol/l (high) equates to a real reading of 4-5 mmol/l (normal) of glucose.

How to go PK if you are already diabetic

Insulin resistance is the hallmark of type 2 diabetes – insulin levels are chronically high because cells become less and less responsive to it as they struggle to maintain normal blood sugar levels in the face of high sugar and starch consumption. When the body loses the fight to maintain normal blood sugar levels, the symptoms of type 2 diabetes result. If not already in ketosis, fasting empties glycogen stores in the liver and muscles (see page 24), reverses insulin resistance and is the quickest way to lose weight, reverse metabolic syndrome and diabetes.

Diabetics and their doctors are naturally anxious about low blood sugar. This can *only* happen if the diabetic person is taking prescribed medication to lower their blood sugar. The key is to monitor blood sugar closely and, as levels come down as they inevitably will, reduce the dose of medication. Type 2 diabetics should be able to stop all medication. Type I diabetics *must* use continuous blood sugar monitoring, such as Dexcom. They eventually need a smaller dose of insulin, and a few will end up on no insulin. The 'brittle' diabetics are stabilised.

Dr Ian Lake, an NHS GP and type I diabetic, did a five-day fast. During this, and alongside other keto-adapted athletes including Matthew Pinsent, four-times Olympic champion, he ran 20 miles daily from Stroud to Bristol. His insulin requirements were unchanged.

Doctors always fret about their patients being in ketosis because the only state they know about is **diabetic ketoacidosis** – a dire emergency. Diabetic ketoacidosis occurs when blood sugar is very high. This problem is entirely preventable with careful blood sugar monitoring.

Balancing total calories, protein and carbs

The next step is to balance up total calories needed on a daily basis (your basic metabolic rate), protein and carbohydrates.

Total calories needed per day

You can calculate what this should be (see below) or look up the recommended calories for your age, weight, height and activity level. Many people who are overweight think they can lose weight through calorie restriction. However, if you eat less than the recommended calorie total for more than a few days, your body will simply switch off calorie burning, making you tired, foggy, cold and depressed. If you are overweight, then the strategy is to first get PK adapted, as above, then to sort out the underactive thyroid (see Chapter 7) and then do the 5:2 diet (see below, page 35, and also our book *Paleo-Ketogenic: The Why and the How*).

Protein – not too little, not too much

Proteins include meat, eggs, fish and shellfish. These are zero carb *but*, if eaten in excess, the body can convert them into sugars. A rule of thumb is to allow 0.7 to 0.9 g of protein per pound (0.45 kg) of lean body mass for protein leverage.

As I have said, the PK diet is not a high-protein diet. It is a high-fat and high-fibre diet (relative to Western diets). Fibre is important to satisfy the appetite. The key is to eat no refined or processed foods and to calculate your protein needs.

Protein leverage

The body cannot store protein, but daily protein is essential for survival. We have a protein appetite which will make us crave food until that appetite has been satisfied. If you are eating a low-protein diet, you will be driven to eat more food. In that process you will overeat carbs and fat, so expect to gain weight. Conversely, eat a high-protein diet and you tend to undereat and lose weight. You need to get your protein intake right to help maintain a normal weight. (Note a high-protein diet is not desirable as the body then has to deal with the toxic consequences of too much protein. Listen to your body and appetite; they will tell you how much you need.)

How to calculate your basic metabolic rate (BMR) and calorie requirements

There are many equations to calculate your BMR (your calorie needs at rest), and from there your calorie needs. We shall be using a tried and tested formula for the BMR, the Mifflin-St Jeor Equations which are:

For Men:
BMR = 10 x weight in kg PLUS 6.25 x height in cm MINUS 5 x age in years PLUS 5
For Women:
BMR = 10 x weight in kg PLUS 6.25 x height in cm MINUS 5 x age years MINUS 161

If you'd rather not do the maths, this handy online calculator does it for you: www.calculator.net/bmr-calculator.html

You will then need to multiply up your BMR (as calculated above) by these factors depending on your level of activity. Again, the website above does this for you:

Sedentary: calories required = BMR x 1.2
Lightly active: calories required = BMR x 1.375
Moderately active (moderate exercise 3-5 days): calories required = BMR x 1.55
Very active (hard exercise 6-7 days a week): calories required = BMR x 1.725
Super-active (hard exercise and sport and physical job): calories required = BMR x 1.9

Table 4.1 gives a worked example based on me.

Table 4.1: Calorie needs at rest (BMR) and when active

Steps **FIRST work out your BMR at rest**	**Worked example** **My vital statistics are:** **Weight 61 kg, height 168 cm, age 62**	**Result for me**
For women: BMR = 10 x weight (kg) PLUS 6.25 x height (cm) minus 5 x age (years) MINUS 161	10 x 61 kg = 610 PLUS 6.25 x 168 cm = 1050 MINUS 5 x 62 = 310 MINUS 161	610 PLUS 1050 MINUS 310 MINUS 161 My BMR is 1189 kcal
For men: BMR = 10 x weight (kg) PLUS 6.25 x height (cm) MINUS 5 x age (years) PLUS 5	Ditto above THEN ADD 5	If I were male, and Craig says I do have balls, the calculation would be: 610 PLUS 1050 MINUS 310 PLUS 5 My BMR would be 1355 kcal
THEN multiply your resting BMR by your activity factor to get your total energy expenditure: • Sedentary x 1.2 • Lightly active x 1.375 • Moderately active (moderate exercise 3-5 days) x 1.55 • Very active (hard exercise 6-7 days a week) x 1.725 • Super-active (hard exercise and sport and physical job) x 1.9	I am moderately active so I: MULTIPLY my BMR by a factor of 1.55 = 1189 x 1.55 = 1843	So my daily energy expenditure is 1843 kcal

Table 4.2: How to calculate your protein requirement

Steps	Worked example – me	Result for me
FIRST work out your daily energy expenditure as above	My daily energy expenditure is 1843 kcal	
Then divide by 4 to give your daily protein need in grams (this need includes recycled protein from self)	DIVIDE 1843 by 4 = 461	
Then adjust for age protein requirements as % of daily energy requirement • Baby to adolescent: 15% • Young adult to 30 years: 18% • Pregnancy and breastfeeding: 20% • 30s: 17% • 40-60: 15% • 60-65: 18% • >65: 20%	I am 62 so I need my diet to be 18% protein 461 x 18/100 = 83	So, I need 83 grams of protein a day

Table 4.3: What and how much to eat to satisfy your protein requirement

Food	Protein content in grams (g) per 100 g	On the plate looks like… approx.	What I eat	My protein consumption approx
Eggs	13	Two eggs	Breakfast: 2 eggs	13
Beef	26	A medium beef burger		
Pork	31	Small pork chop	Supper, main course: pork chop	31
Bacon	Up to 39 depending on how fatty; 1 slice = 8 g			

Table 4.3: *Cont'd*

Food	Protein content in grams (g) per 100 g	On the plate looks like… approx.	What I eat	My protein consumption approx
Lamb	26	One lamb chop		
Chicken, duck	20 27	Whole breast or Whole leg		
Fish, fresh	29	A good chunk		
Prawns	25	A prawn 'cocktail' starter	Supper, starters: paté or fish	25
Brazil nuts	15		Snacks	10-15
				My total: 79-84

Once you have things roughly balanced out your body will do the rest. Appetite and desire for food are remarkably accurate once you have addiction out of the way. Interestingly, before I did this calculation, what's listed in Table 4.3 was what I ate, so my brain and body had worked it out already.

If the PK diet does not suit

If the PK diet really does not suit in the short term, this may be due to a detox and die-off (DDD) reaction (see Appendix 2) or to ketogenic hypoglycaemia associated with an underactive thyroid (Chapter 7).

If the PK diet really does not suit in the long term: We do know that sugar is a vital part of metabolism, *not* as a fuel, but as a building block to make DNA and RNA. It is also essential for detoxing via the glucuronide pathway in the liver. I am happy for carbs to come into the diet so long as you are in ketosis at least once a day. I think the most important information is that being in ketosis tells us our glycogen stores are squeezed dry. At this point, consuming some carbs is fine – if you slip out of ketosis for a short time then you are doing no harm. I am sometimes out of ketosis in the morning, but by late afternoon I am invariably blowing ketones.

Sugars may come from protein (via gluconeogenesis) or of course from eating carbs. Low protein and zero carb diets are not desirable, as already explained.

If you really struggle to get into ketosis, then I suggest the 5:2 diet (see our book *Paleo-Ketogenic: The Why and the How*). This means you eat as low-carb as you can manage for five days, and then for two days a week you eat a very low-carb, or possibly carnivore, diet, or possibly fast until you get into ketosis. The important point here is that to get into ketosis you have to squeeze dry the hitherto saturated glycogen 'sponges' in the liver and muscles. Once these have been emptied, blood sugar control is much easier as the body is not relying on insulin for such. The blood sugar spikes and dips are ironed out.

What is right for you

Remember that the above are not hard and fast rules. Listen to your body and follow your appetite. Once you are not addicted to any foods, this is a remarkably good guide:

> *Variety is the very spice of life, that gives it all its flavour.*
>
> *The Task* by William Cowper (1785)

Change your diet with the seasons and through life. Eat the non-addictive foods that you enjoy most because these will be the very foods that you need. A wide variety of foods will grow a wide variety of microbes in the gut. Include as many spices and herbs as you can. Taste has evolved for excellent reasons. Eat foods that are minimally processed. If you can, become a gardener and grow your own. My garden holds a special place in my heart, and if you are lucky enough to have space to grow things, and are physically capable, then do give it a go. It is highly likely that you, too, will grow to love your garden – you will be in good company.

> *If you have a garden and a library, you have everything you need.*
>
> *Ad Familiares*, Letter IV to Varro by Marcus Tullius Cicero
> (3 January 106 BC – 7 December 43 BC)

However many years she lived, Mary always felt that 'she should never forget that first morning when her garden began to grow'.

The Secret Garden by Frances Hodgson Burnett
(24 November 1849 – 29 October 1924)

My garden is my most beautiful masterpiece.

Claude Monet, French Impressionist painter
(14 November 1840 – 5 December 1926)

The greatest fine art of the future will be the making of a comfortable living from a small piece of land.

Abraham Lincoln, US President (12 February 1809 – 15 April 1865)

You can see me in action in my garden in these YouTube videos:
www.youtube.com/watch?v=B8ZKYSWW_VI
www.youtube.com/watch?v=gI4yzqRp5as

Timing – when to eat

Primitive man did not eat three regular meals a day, neither did he need to snack. Consultant neurologist Dale Bredesen reverses dementia with a PK diet[3] but insists all daily food be consumed within a 10-hour window of time. These days I eat lunch and supper within a seven-hour window.

Once keto-adapted you may feel a bit peckish and deserving of a snack, but the good news is that you will not get the associated 'energy dive' experienced by the carb addict who must eat according to the clock. Carb addicts experience a sudden loss of energy and *have* to feed their addiction to get rid of this awful feeling. The keto-adapted do not experience this so long as thyroid function is normal (see Chapter 7). A weekly 24-hour fast is also good for the metabolism. It may be counterintuitive, but the fact is that this enhances mental and physical performance.

If you have decided to go ahead with this diet, and you *really* should, then believe me it is a bumpy ride. There is a whole new language to be learned. You will have to identify the 'glycogen sponge', anticipate the initial worsening of withdrawal symptoms and 'keto 'flu', get 'keto-adapted' and prepare for diet, die-off and detox (DDD) reactions (see Appendix 2). I simply cannot write all the extensive detail here for this successful transition without losing the plot of this book. So at least get our book *Paleo-Ketogenic: The Why and the How*, which will hold your intellectual hand through this difficult transition. Or just do it!

Once established on the PK diet

The word 'doctor' comes from the Latin 'to teach'. I can show you the path, but you have to walk it. You have to become your own doctor. All diagnosis starts with hypothesis. We know the PK diet is the starting point to treat every disease and that is non-negotiable. Stick with this diet for life and it may be that this is all you have to do. Once PK is established you have to ask if you are functioning to your full physical and mental potential. Only you can know this.

If you are functioning to your full potential, then you can take the occasional liberty with your diet. Primitive man surely did. He did so in the autumn, although not with the high-carb foods that we can now access. He would have feasted on fruit for this autumnal period. Alcohol is a peculiar problem – it is addictive, high-carb and stimulates insulin directly. But I love alcohol – the jokes are so much funnier with a glass of cider on board – and so I enjoy this occasional liberty at this stage in my life. I have to because Craig keeps sending me bottles of the most delicious cider… and I do not have the will power to tell him to stop… (Craig replies, 'Then I shall carry on… luckily in return, I get delicious joints of pork and bacon…'.)

If you are not functioning to your full potential, then you must stick with the PK diet and read on. Even if you do not experience immediate benefits you will greatly increase your chance of a long and healthy life. It is a great consolation for me to be able to tell my CFS, ME and LC patients that their best years are ahead of them.

The Chinese do not draw any distinction between food and medicine.

Lin Yutang, Chinese writer (1895 – 1976) in
The importance of Living, chapter 9, section 7

THE UPPER FERMENTING GUT

The second step in putting the basics in place is to tackle the upper fermenting gut. The human gut is almost unique in the mammalian world. The upper gut (the first 20 feet (c 6 metres) of oesophagus, stomach, duodenum, jejunum and ileum) is a sterile carnivorous gut (like a dog's) designed for digesting protein and fat. The lower gut (the last 3 feet (c 1 metre) of colon is a fermenting vegetarian gut designed to utilise fibre (like a horse except humans cannot ferment that toughest fibre, cellulose). This allows humans to deal with many different foods and partly explains our success as a species.

This system works perfectly until we overwhelm our ability to deal with sugars and starches by consuming these too much and/or too often. Bacteria and yeasts then move in to colonise the hitherto sterile upper gut and start fermenting any available carbohydrates. This includes the condition small bowel bacterial overgrowth (SIBO); the bacterium that causes stomach and duodenal ulcers – *Helicobacter pylori*; 'candida' overgrowth; some parasites and any other microbes that should not be present. This scenario is what I call the upper fermenting gut (UFG), and it is bad news. Why? Because it creates nasty symptoms and pathology including:

1. Foods are fermented to toxins such as ethyl, propyl and butyl alcohols, D lactate, ammonia compounds, hydrogen, hydrogen sulphide and much else. This fermentation is otherwise known as the 'auto-brewery syndrome'. All these nasties have the potential to poison us, and symptoms of this include foggy brain. I just need a glass of wine to appreciate that fact!
2. Colonies of bacteria and fungi build up and are then further colonised by viruses (so-called bacteriophages). Fermenting microbes produce bacterial endotoxin, fungal mycotoxins and viral particles.
3. These toxins spill over into the portal vein and so to the liver. The liver uses up a lot of energy and raw materials to deal with them. This is debilitating.

4. The gases generated by upper gut fermentation cause borborygmi (gut rumbling), burping and bloating. They may distend the gut, and this is painful.
5. Microbes move into the lining of the gut and this low-grade inflammation results in leaky gut. This means that acid cannot be concentrated in the stomach because it leaks out as fast as it is secreted in. Acid is an essential part of digestion because:
6. i) it is essential to start the digestion of protein.
   ii) it is necessary to absorb minerals.
   iii) it sterilises the upper gut and protects us from infections.
   iv) it determines gut emptying. An insufficiently acid stomach does not empty correctly and this drives reflux, oesophagitis, heartburn and hiatus hernia.
7. Microbes, dead and alive, and undigested foods leak into the bloodstream and drive pathology at distal sites. This is a major cause of pathology from inflammatory bowel disease, arthritis, fibromyalgia, connective tissue disease, autoimmunity, interstitial cystitis, urticaria, venous ulcers, intrinsic asthma, kidney disease, and possibly psychosis and other brain pathologies such as Parkinson's disease.
8. Chronic inflammation of the lining of the gut results in cancer, especially of the stomach and oesophagus. Both are on the increase. Diet is the main reason, followed by acid blocking drugs such as proton pump inhibitors (PPIs) that are massively over-prescribed for long-term use. These drugs also drive osteoporosis.

Fermentation of fibre by friendly microbes should take place in the colon – that is, the lower gut. The gases which result and make you fart are hydrogen and methane. These farts are odourless. Put a match to them and they will explode… not that I recommend this even for diagnostic purposes! If your farts are offensive, then that is because you have overwhelmed your digestion upstream and proteins are being fermented in your colon – rotting meat stinks. Short gut transit time will have a similar effect. Professor Gibson, a food microbiologist from the University of Reading with an impressive research CV,[4] divides people into 'inflammables' and 'smellies' – the inflammables (hydrogen and methane) have normal gut fermentation and the smellies (hydrogen sulphide) do not.[†]

Getting rid of the upper fermenting gut

Getting rid of the UFG is easy. Remember it includes all types of fermentation – small intestinal bacterial overgrowth (SIBO), for example. The steps are:

- Starve out the fermenting microbes with a PK diet. They need starches and sugars to live on and without these they cannot survive.
- Kill 'em with vitamin C (5 g or go to bowel intolerance as described on page 44, in the morning/during the day) and Lugol's iodine 15% (3 drops at night). Both contact-kill all microbes and are amongst my favourite multitasking tools.
- Remember to take vitamin C and iodine at least 2 hours apart. Vitamin C is a reducing agent – it donates electrons to neutralise toxic free radicals. Iodine is an oxidising agent – it accepts electrons to neutralise free radicals. Taken together they thus can cancel each other out.
- Give it time. You never completely sterilise the gut – the idea is to keep numbers so low that the odd carb feast does not matter. Given the right substrate, microbes double their numbers every 20 minutes – they grow exponentially. If one just has a few thousand microbes, then after hours of freely available food there will only be a few million microbes, which cause no problem – the immune system can deal with this. However, if the baseline is a few million, then a carb feast will grow billions and that does overwhelm the immune system to drive inflammation.
- Then, take the Basic Package and perhaps add in intermittent fasting in which daily food is consumed within a six-hour window of time.

†**Note from Craig:** At my secondary school, Aylesbury Grammar School, the prevailing odour indicated that most boys were smellies. However, one boy, in my class, was capable of, and regularly demonstrated at house parties and in the sports changing rooms, his ability to light his own farts. We all considered this a gift from the Gods, a super-power! It is only now that I have put two and two together and realised that this boy went home for lunch where baked beans were his staple – lots of fibre which he fermented to inflammable methane and hydrogen in his lower gut.

SUPPLEMENTS: THE BASIC PACKAGE

The word 'supplement' derives from the Latin *supplementum* ('that which is added to supply a shortage') and so describes exactly what is happening – we need to give our bodies minerals and vitamins because these are in short supply due to our modern methods of growing food.

What I call the 'Basic Package' is essential because at the present time there is a one-way movement of minerals from soil to plants to animals to humans and then into our rivers and seas. Minerals are not recycled. Without minerals, plants and our microbiomes cannot synthesise vitamins. This is compounded by glyphosate, the most widely used herbicide, which is a chelating agent. It kills plants by binding minerals up in soil, so depriving them of vital nutrients. Worse still, glyphosate is used to kill unwanted plants ('weeds') just before harvesting so any minerals that do remain are further sequestered. To help compensate for these inevitable deficiencies we all need the Basic Package, vis:

- A multivitamin with 25 mg of the common B vitamins.
- Sunshine salt[‡] – I put this together because I could not find a mineral preparation with all the essential minerals, in good doses, in a soluble form and in the correct proportions. (See Useful resources, page 303.)
- Essential fatty acids – A tablespoon of hemp oil. Alternatively, evening primrose oil and fish oils.
- Vitamin D 10,000 iu daily (approximately equivalent to one hour of sunshine).
- Vitamin C 5 g or go to your bowel tolerance (morning/during the day). Use vitamin C to help cure the upper fermenting gut. In the early days of tackling this problem, many people need much higher doses. Once you have sorted it out, your dose of vitamin C should not cause any gut symptoms.

[‡]**Sunshine salt:** I have got to the stage of my medicine where I know exactly what must be done so I am now trying to make this as easy and inexpensive as possible. So, I have put together Sunshine Salt, which contains all essential minerals from sodium and selenium to magnesium and manganese together with vitamins D 5000 iu and B12 5 mg in a 5-g (1 tsp) dose. This does make life much easier. It tastes like a slightly piquant sea salt, can be used in cooking and means the rest of the family get a dose without realising it.

Taking vitamin C to bowel tolerance

Ascorbic acid (AA) is the best and the cheapest form of vitamin C. I suggest using the powder form and adding this to your daily bottle of water, so that it is consumed little and often through the day – but do take vitamin C away from Iodine as they work in different ways and can 'cancel' each other out (see more detail in Appendix 1: Groundhog Chronic).

Start with 2 g and build up by 1 g a day until you start to get gut symptoms. The idea is that vitamin C arrives in the upper gut and contact-kills all fermenters there. The body absorbs what it needs for other functions: good antioxidant status, detoxing, dealing with systemic infection, killing cancer cells and more. Any vitamin C surplus to requirements remains in the gut and passes into the large bowel. Here, it will start to kill some of the friendly fermenters, which are then fermented by other friendlies to produce gurgling and offensive farts. Increasing the dose further causes diarrhoea. Gurgling and farts will do nicely to indicate you have arrived at bowel tolerance. Then reduce the dose to just below that unsociable dose at which gurgling, and farts are produced. This is *your* bowel tolerance level and will differ from person to person but usually is about 5 g per day.

The dose may change with age and circumstance. With an acute infection it can increase to 100 g or more depending on the infection. The moment you get an acute infection, take 10 g AA every hour until you reach your bowel tolerance. You determine where your bowel tolerance is in exactly the same way as described above – that is, by reference to that dose at which the gurgling and farts occur – your bowel tolerance is just below that dose. See our book, *The Infection Game* for much more detail.

If AA is not tolerated, then add magnesium carbonate ($MgCO_3$); two parts AA to one part $MgCO_3$, by weight (e.g. 2 grams to 1 gram), results in a non-acidic, neutral solution. This also gives you a good dose of magnesium. Once you are PK- and vitamin C-adapted you should tolerate AA well.

PRACTICALITIES

Table 4.4: Overview and fine-tuning of the PK diet lifestyle

Dietary issue (good or bad)	**Why?**	**What to do**
Addiction to sugar, fruit, caffeine, alcohol, nicotine, cannabis	Addiction masks appetite and we consume for all the wrong reasons. Addictions disturb sleep quality and quantity. Addictions mask symptoms. One addiction switches on the others	Use addictions occasionally and in moderation
Most Westerners are carbohydrate addicts	Too much carbohydrate drives pathology: fatigue, obesity, high blood pressure, diabetes, cancer, arteriosclerosis and dementia ('type 3 diabetes')	Get into ketosis – use the ketone breath meter to demonstrate such. In ketosis your muscle and liver glycogen sponges are squeezed dry. That means the body can easily deal with any carbs in the diet
	If you overwhelm the ability of the upper gut to digest, then it will ferment and that drives even more pathology. Symptoms include: gastritis, reflux, GORD, bloating, burping and foggy brain. Pathology includes: fatigue, inflammation, autoimmunity, toxicity and much more	Do not over-eat carbs. Take vitamin C to bowel tolerance. Take Lugol's iodine 15% 2-3 drops at night. Fast
Some carbo-hydrate is fine	Sugars are needed as building blocks (to make DNA, RNA and ATP) and to detox (glucuronidation), but not too much. The body can make sugar from proteins	Use the ketone breath meter to monitor how you flip in and out of ketosis – that makes sure you are not over-loading with carbs. Get your carbs from vegetables, nuts and seeds. If you never blow positive for ketones, fast until you get a positive test result. If you still struggle then this points to the ketogenic hypoglycaemia of the underactive thyroid (see Chapter 7)

Table 4.4: *Cont'd*

Dietary issue (good or bad)	Why?	What to do
Fats are highly desirable	As fuel – the keto-adapted athlete performs 7-15% better. As building blocks for all cells, including mitochondria (our energy powerhouses). Fats are especially needed for building brain and immune system cells	Eat fatty meat, fish, poultry, duck, eggs, butter. Lard, dripping, goose fat, coconut oil are ideal for cooking. Oils must not be heated (or you create toxic trans fats)
Dairy products are meant for young mammals	Too much is a risk for cancer, heart disease, osteoporosis	Cut out all dairy products. The safest dairy products are butter and ghee. Vegan butters, cheeses, coconut milks and coconut yoghurts make good replacements
Western diets are low in fibre	Fibre makes for chewing which stimulates digestion. Fibre is essential for the friendly fermentation in the large bowel to produce fuel (short chain fatty acids), vitamins (B and K) and bulk for effortless passage of stool. Friendly fermentation programmes the immune system and protects against infection	Eat sufficient fibre until you pass a Bristol stool chart number 4, once or twice daily effortlessly, ideally using a squatty potty. Make the PK linseed bread which is 24% fibre, 2% carb (see our book *Paleo-Ketogenic: The Why and the How*)
Processed food is generally high in carbs and low in nutrients	Is often addictive (high-carb, low-protein), deficient in micronutrients, toxic with chemicals, low in fibre. Some define processed food as any product having more than five ingredients	Do not eat processed food – eat real food
Eat as varied a diet as possible	We know that the more diverse the microbes of the gut the healthier. Each microbe has a liking for a certain food	Keep ringing the changes and eat foods that are in season
	Once you have conquered addiction your body and brain will tell you what and how much to eat. You have separate appetites for protein, fat, carbs, salt, micronutrients and possibly more	Listen to your appetite – if you fancy it you probably need it

Dietary issue (good or bad)	Why?	What to do
	If we become ill, we develop an appetite for healing herbs, essential oils and other remedies. This is well established in animals and is called zoopharmacognosy.[§] Humans are also animals	Listen to your appetite, brain and body. When ill, it may tell you to fast and sniff
Make sure you are eating sufficient calories	Many people half-starve themselves in a misguided attempt to lose weight. This simply makes you tired, cold, foggy-brained and depressed	Use the Mifflin St Jeor Equations equation (above) to work out your daily need
Vitamin C deficiency is pandemic	Humans have lost the ability to synthesise vitamin C from sugars	Take vitamin C as ascorbic acid. Everyone's dose is different: take to bowel tolerance or to urine tolerance (test with vitamin C urine test strips[¶]) Most need 5-8 g (5000-8000 mg) daily, much more for acute infections
Micronutrient deficiencies are pandemic	Soils are depleted by modern agriculture and lack of recycling of human compost back to the soils	Take a good multivitamin daily and Sunshine Salt 5 g AND essential fatty acids (in the Basic Package as above)
Allergies are common	Irritable bowel, headaches, asthma, arthritis are often allergy driven	Cut out common allergens e.g. dairy, gluten and yeast. Cut out known allergens

[§]**Linguistic note:** The word 'zoo pharmacognosy' derives from the Greek roots *zoo* ('animal'), *pharmacon* ('drug, medicine') and *gnosy* ('knowing'). I loved Caroline Ingraham's book *Animal Self-Medication*, which is full of information and wonderful case histories – we should all learn from case histories. Interested readers are also referred to *Really Wild Remedies—Medicinal Plant Use by Animals* by Jennifer A Biser of the Smithsonian National Zoological Park, USA .[5]

[¶]**Footnote:** Vitamin C urine test stripsare readily available online – see Useful resources, page 303.

Table 4.4: *Cont'd*

Dietary issue (good or bad)	Why?	What to do
Protein is essential on a daily basis	Protein leverage: Too little protein in the diet will stimulate the appetite to eat any food (often high-carb foods) until the protein appetite is satisfied. Overeating calories causes obesity	Calculate your protein requirement as above
Food being constantly present in the upper gut	This means the stomach never has a chance to heal, repair and restore normal stomach acidity	Eat all food within a 7-10-hour window of time. Do not snack. Early supper improves sleep quality
Food being constantly present in the mouth	This means the mouth never has a chance to heal, repair and reduce numbers of bacteria. Bacterial overgrowth leads to gum disease and tooth decay	Ditto above
Fasting has great benefits	Primitive man did not eat three meals a day. Fasting switches on autophagy which protects against cancer and degeneration. It switches on stem cells for the new growth and repair. Fasting clears the foggy brain. Fasting squeezes dry the glycogen sponge and gets you into ketosis rapidly	Do a 24-hour fast weekly (e.g. skip breakfast and lunch for one day a week). Do a 48-hour fast monthly. Perhaps do longer fasting once a year
Exercise	Do the right sort of daily anaerobic exercise to increase muscle bulk. This keeps you strong and increases your BMR. (See Chapter 9: Exercise)	With more muscle you need to eat more. Jolly good – I love food and I am greedy!

Summary

This is a long chapter but can be summarised briefly.

- Do the PK diet – this is non-negotiable. Measure ketones to make sure you are in ketosis.
- If you are highly allergic, you may have to begin with the carnivore diet.
- If you struggle despite being in ketosis, check thyroid function (see Chapter 7).
- If you wish to lose weight, do not restrict calories but do the 5:2 diet.
- Get rid of any upper fermenting gut problems with the PK diet, vitamin C to bowel tolerance and iodine.
- After ridding yourself of any fermenting gut issues, take the Basic Package of supplements as listed in this chapter. Take it for life.
- Consider intermittent fasting: consuming all food within a daily six-hour window of time.
- If you are already diabetic, still do the PK diet but do re-read the relevant section above.
- Finetune the PK diet as you get better.
- This may be all you need to do. If you feel you are living life to its full potential after putting in place the PK diet, ridding yourself of any fermenting gut issues and taking the Basic Package, then you are done. Carry on with the PK diet and Basic Package for life.

Chapter 5

It's mitochondria, not hypochondria

This chapter is based on my clinical work and the three research studies that it gave rise to. These studies provide the evidence base for this book – that CFS, ME and long Covid arise from mitochondria (the little engines found inside almost every cell in the body) not fulfilling their role as generators of all the energy we need.

For those who wish to fully understand the results of my published research findings, there is only one way – read them.[1, 2, 3] But, as I have said, this book is written on a 'need to know' basis and so what follows gives enough for you to understand what the papers concluded and, more importantly, what this means for treatment. Here are the details of my three published papers, and I pay tribute to my co-authors, Professor Norman Booth and Dr John McLaren-Howard, without whom these papers would neither have been written nor published.

- 16th January 2009 saw the publication of 'Chronic fatigue syndrome and mitochondrial dysfunction'. The paper was published in the *International Journal of Clinical and Experimental Medicine*. The full text of the paper can be accessed from the link in the reference list.[1]
- Our second paper, 'Mitochondrial dysfunction and the pathophysiology of Myalgic Encephalomyelitis/Chronic Fatigue Syndrome (ME/CFS)', was published in the *International Journal of Clinical and Experimental Medicine* on 30 June 2012.[2]
- November 2012 saw the publication of our third paper entitled 'Targeting mitochondrial dysfunction in the treatment of Myalgic Encephalomyelitis/Chronic Fatigue Syndrome (ME/CFS) – a clinical audit'.[3]

I consider dysfunctional mitochondria to be the central pathophysiological lesion – that is, the underlying physical problem – where there is chronic fatigue, because all other lesions manifest on or via mitochondria. That is to say, and as explained in Chapter 2, all symptoms associated with CFS are explicable by assuming mitochondrial failure. Mitochondria are the common engines that power all eukaryotic cells (organisms whose cells contain a nucleus and other membrane-bound organelles), in animals and plants, bacteria and fungi, indeed effectively in all life forms (bar prokaryotes ('archaea' and some bacteria) and a few rare exceptions). They are the powerhouse of the cell – the electrical energy gradients they generate across cell membranes are similar to those within bolts of lightning. Altogether, 30% of heart muscle is comprised of mitochondria and each heart cell contains up to 2000 of these micro-structures. Their main function is to generate the energy molecule ATP and this they do with remarkable efficiency. A molecule can be recycled every 10 seconds. However, their extraordinary complexities mean they are highly susceptible to vagaries in their environment. They have to be looked after and not abused but Western diets and lifestyles are killing the very life force within us.

All medical students learn about mitochondria, but then they forget about them. That happened in my day because conventional medicine ignored them and gave them no clinical application. It still does! I loved biochemistry because it was so logical. I cherished the work of Peter Mitchell, a cattle farmer in Cornwall, who won the Nobel Prize in 1978 for his discovery of the mechanism by which mitochondria generated energy (ATP) from fuel and oxygen.

In his speech at the Nobel Banquet on 10 December 1978, Peter Mitchell said that: 'The final outcome cannot be known, either to the originator of a new theory, or to his colleagues and critics, who are bent on falsifying it. Thus, the scientific innovator may feel all the more lonely and uncertain.' And indeed, it took over 20 years for others to realise that mitochondria are implicated in nearly all disease processes, from diabetes and dementia, cancer and coronaries to autism and arthritis. This makes perfect biological sense—if you impair energy delivery to any organ, then it will fail. If mitochondria do not work properly, then the energy supply to every cell in the body will be impaired. The variation in degrees of failure explains the wide range of symptoms and pathologies.

During my first 20 years of NHS work, from the 1980s to 2000, I had seen some modest successes treating CFS and ME sufferers using all the tools of the trade that I knew at that time to be effective, such as diet, supplements, pacing, correcting thyroid function and so on. However, I was left with a hard core of patients who were no better, and I was still scrambling around for answers. I am inquisitive and hate to be beaten – ask my Team Chase colleagues.* All the time, I felt the need to understand more, and I forever had the words of Robert Boyle, the famous scientist (25 January 1627 – 31 December 1691) who originated Boyle's Law, ringing in my ears: 'It is highly dishonourable for a reasonable soul to live in so divinely built a mansion as the body she resides in - altogether unacquainted with the exquisite structure of it.'†

In my quest, I had the services of neither Newton nor Boyle to hand, but I was extraordinarily fortunate to find an intellectual equivalent in John McLaren-Howard. He was the biochemical genius that I needed to address some of the difficult biochemical questions that I had. Without John's generosity, skill and expertise I would still be stuck in the 20th century.

Clinically, patients with severe CFS looked like my patients with heart failure. This makes perfect sense – if mitochondria go slow, cells go slow, and organs go slow. The heart is a pump and in CFS it does not have the energy to beat powerfully and therefore cardiac output falls. This has been confirmed by work by Dr Arnold Peckerman.

Dr Peckerman was asked by the US National Institutes of Health to develop a test for CFS in order to help them to judge the level of disability in patients claiming Social Security benefits. He is a cardiologist and on the basis that CFS patients suffer low blood pressure, low blood volume and perfusion defects, he surmised that they were in

*__Sporting note from Craig:__ Team chasing is a cross-country event with rider and horse trying to complete a set course in the shortest time. Various penalties can occur and it is a *very* competitive and *high* adrenaline sport. Sarah has cracked her skull three times doing this! Those who wish to know more, please see: www.horse-events.co.uk/events/team-chasing/

†**Historical note:** Sir Isaac Newton (25 December 1642 – 20 March 1726/27) corresponded with Boyle and one such letter, written in 1679, has been put online: www.orgonelab.org/newtonletter.htm In summary, Newton says of Boyle: 'For my own part, I have so little fancy to things of this nature, that had not your encouragement moved me to it, I should never, I think, have thus far set pen to paper about them.' Praise indeed!

a low cardiac output state. He measured cardiac output using impedance cardiography and concluded his results in his paper of 2003.[4] Furthermore, the level of impairment correlated very closely with the level of disability in patients:

> *Results: The patients with severe CFS had significantly lower stroke volume and cardiac output than the controls and less ill patients. Post exertional fatigue and flu-like symptoms of infection differentiated the patients with severe CFS from those with less severe CFS (88.5% concordance) and were predictive (R2 = 0.46, P < 0.0002) of lower cardiac output. In contrast, neuropsychiatric symptoms showed no specific association with cardiac output.*

My CFS patients were not in heart failure for any of the usual reasons such as poor blood supply, death of heart tissue following infarctions (blocked blood vessels), leaky valves or pacemaker problems. There had to be another reason. What about mitochondria? 'Dear John,' went my letter, 'I need a test of mitochondrial function. Please can you arrange this as soon as possible.' Poor man – this must have kept him sleepless for weeks!

Initially he measured the activity of individual enzymes within mitochondria, including the complexes I to V which drove the process of chemiosmosis identified by Nobel-Prize-winning Peter Mitchell. (Put briefly, this is the movement of ions across a semipermeable-membrane-bound structure, down their electrochemical gradient.) We could not see any clear correlation with the level of energy in my patients. (Interestingly, the best correlation was with levels of NAD (vitamin B3). This is the most important intermediary between Krebs citric acid cycle and chemiosmosis.) I stamped my little foot and pursed my lips in a petulant way. 'I don't care about the complexes. I want a functional test, John. I want something that tells us about how ATP is produced. Get back to that drawing board.'[‡]

Thankfully John's tolerance parallels his brilliance and innovative skills. There are many tests in research biochemistry that are not used clinically because they are perceived to have no medical application. John's forte is to single out and further develop tests

[‡]I feel rather put out that Sarah has never stamped her little foot at me! Craig

which do have clinical application – he ploughs his own furrow. In this respect he has developed a wide range of clinically relevant and applicable tests. But what he developed at the time were the revolutionary mitochondrial function tests which started with 'ATP profiles'.

What we learned from 'ATP profiles'

What did we learn from John McLaren-Howard's mitochondrial function tests? A lot, as described next. This is based on the publication of the three peer-reviewed scientific papers listed above, 1036 ATP profiles, and the patients I dealt with, together with over two decades of my own clinical experience and that of many colleagues. The importance of this wealth of knowledge is that it is not essential to have mitochondrial function tests performed in order to recover. We know by now that the regimes described in this book are highly effective.

We learned that:

1. Those with the worst levels of fatigue had the worst mitochondrial function. You can see this from the graph in our first paper (reproduced here as Figure 5.1). It is self-explanatory. Thank you, Professor Norman Booth of Mansfield College Oxford, for writing this up and thank you Craig for the number crunching and graphs. Sadly Norman Booth died in 2018, but his legacy lives on in this work and also the many other papers that he had a hand in publishing – 158 to be precise.[5]
2. John also measured micronutrients known to be vital for mitochondrial function – namely, magnesium, coenzyme Q10, niacinamide (vitamin B3 or NAD), acetyl-L-carnitine, levels of ATP, glutathione peroxidase (selenium and glutathione), mitochondrial superoxide (manganese dependent), intracellular and extracellular superoxide dismutase (zinc and manganese dependent). He measured how well energy was released in the conversion of ATP to ADP in the cell (a magnesium-dependent process). This allowed us to work out the package of nutritional supplements necessary to correct deficiencies of processes that are easily blocked. John developed further tests of translocator protein function to see what exactly was blocking these processes.
3. He also measured:

Figure 5.1: Graph showing the relationship between CFS patients' scores for abnormal factors and scores for mitochondrial energy, from my first paper.[1]

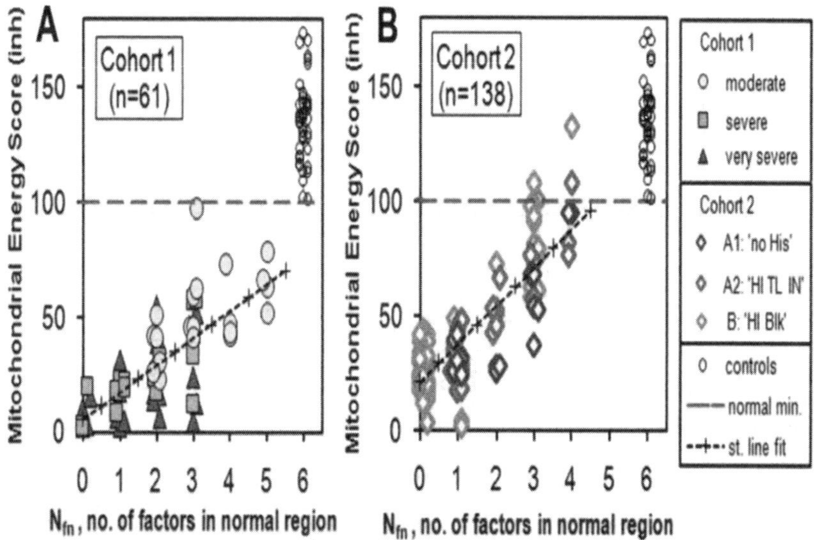

(a) the rate of oxidative phosphorylation (put briefly, this is the cellular process that harnesses the reduction of oxygen to generate high-energy phosphate bonds in the form of adenosine triphosphate (ATP), the energy molecule).

(b) how efficiently ATP was exported from mitochondria to the cell (TL IN – this refers to the direction in which TL protein is looking, not the direction that ATP is heading).

(c) how well ADP was recycled back into the mitochondria via translocator protein. (TL OUT – TL is looking out to pull ADP back into mitochondria). This has obvious implications for detoxification regimes.

4. He also did more detailed tests of the rate of oxidative phosphorylation and membrane potentials, which yielded useful information about the matching of energy demand to energy delivery; many showed uncoupling – this is where energy demands and energy delivered are not matched. We now know this may occur with some chemicals, with fructose in its metabolism to uric acid and probably with poor thyroid and adrenal function.

John McLaren-Howard is a genius. He deserves a Nobel Prize for biochemistry. I was lucky to hang on to his coat-tails. As a result of the above tests, we were able to develop tailored regimes for our CFS sufferers. Some went on to have repeat tests and this resulted in our third paper.[3]

Although the numbers were small, the results were astonishingly good – all 30 who did the regimes (those on the left of the graphs in Figure 5.2) improved their mitochondrial function, all four who did not do the regimes (those on the right AX, AV, ZB and AO) worsened their mitochondrial function.

The first columns are the initial tests, the second columns are the follow up after the regimes.

What these graphs tell us is that we can improve mitochondrial function reliably well without tests. This is good news for my PBs (see page xvi). The RBs can get these tests from Professor Koenig in Germany via the Academy of Nutritional Medicine and Armin laboratories (see Useful Resources, page 303) but these are not essential for recovery. I would prefer my PBs to spend their precious resources on the best food they can afford and other such essentials rather than testing.

Figure 5.2: Mitochondrial profile: Initial and follow-up test results for 34 patients

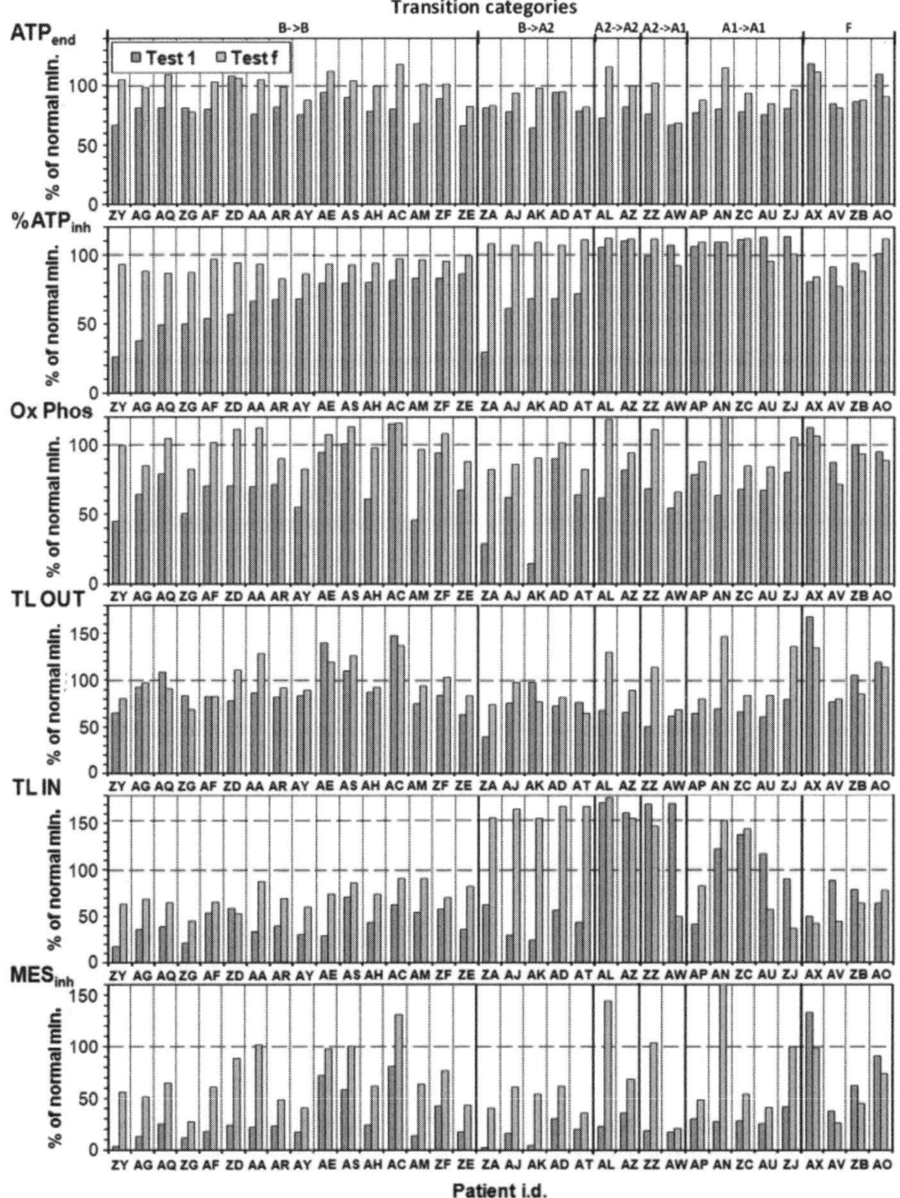

Table 5.1: How to improve the functioning of the mitochondrial engines

What	Why	How
The mitochondrial engines must work and to do this they need the right fuel in the tank	Primarily ketones – yes this is repetition, but this is often the single most important intervention	PK diet
The raw materials to function:	Spark plugs (magnesium)	Magnesium (Mg) 300 mg and vitamin D 10,000 iu for its absorption
	Oil (co-enzyme Q10 and niacinamide)	Co-Q10 100 mg Niacinamide 1500 mg
	Fuel delivery (acetyl-L-carnitine) into mitochondria (which are within cells)	Acetyl-L-carnitine 1 gram (g)
		D-ribose 5-15 g daily – this is the raw material to make de novo ATP – should one really over-do things; helps prevent the post-exertional malaise
Freedom from blocking by:	Lactic acid	Must pace activity – yes, I know this is boring! See Chapter 9
	Toxins from the upper fermenting gut (alcohol, D-lactate, hydrogen sulphide, ammoniacal compounds and many others)	Sort out the upper fermenting gut with a PK diet, vitamin C, 5 g (or to bowel tolerance) by day, and Lugol's iodine 15%, 3 drops at night
	Malondialdehyde and other such from poor antioxidant status	Ketones as a fuel (sugar as a fuel generates free radicals)
		Antioxidants: Co-Q10, superoxide dismutase (zinc 30 mg, manganese 3 mg, copper 1 mg), glutathione peroxidase (selenium 200 mcg, glutathione 250 mg) Vitamin C 5 g
	Social drugs: sugar, alcohol, caffeine, nicotine, chocolate	Addictions are good servants but bad masters. Use very occasionally to enhance a jolly

What	Why	How
	Prescription drugs: the vast majority do not address root causes and accelerate underlying pathology	Work out why you need these (see our book *Ecological Medicine*). Get symptom free and aim to stop them all
	Pesticides and volatile organic compounds	Avoid Get rid of these with heating regimes including: Epsom salt baths; heat from infrared (keeping warm, sunshine, heat belts or lamps) then wash off (see Chapter 14)
	Toxic metals	Avoid. Measure. Get rid of these with chelation and food clays (see Chapter 14)
	Electromagnetic radiation: 5G, mobile phones, cordless phones and wifi – disrupts the electrical potential across all cell membranes	Avoid[6]
Ability to heal and repair	Methylation Sulphation	Methylation – measure homocysteine which should be 5-10 mcmol/l Glutathione 250 mg Vitamin B12 injections (great for the foggy brain) Sulphur as DMSO 20 ml daily
Reduce inflammation	Inflammation increases the friction in the system and blocks mitochondria with inflammatory mediators	Reduce inflammation (see Chapter 13)
Get all the above in the correct 3D position	This requires the 'fourth phase of water'[7]. Also essential for oxygen delivery, which needs good capillary circulation	Heat from infrared (keeping warm, sunshine, heat belts or lamps) DMSO 20 ml daily (See Chapter 13 on reducing inflammation)
Re-educate the mitochondria		Micro-immunotherapy remedies MISEN and MIREG (see Chapter 19 on reprogramming the immune system)

Useful tools of the trade

You can read much more in our book *Ecological Medicine* but all you *need* to know is below. All of these tools are available to all, will multitask, are affordable for my PBs and are intrinsically safe. The potential for harm, other than die-off and detox (DDD) reactions (see Appendix 2), is zero. If you are not sure what to do, then do them all! Start low and build up slow.

Table 5.2: The mitochondrial package – Tools of the trade

Tools	Dose	Their primary job	What they also do
Vitamin C	Aim for 5 g (or to bowel tolerance) daily in the day	Clean up the upper fermenting gut	Essential for antioxidant status (to neutralise free radicals). Bullets with which the immune system kills infections. Anti-inflammatory and anti-allergic. Bind to toxic metals to help excretion. Essential to make adrenal hormones. Essential for connective tissue. Essential for eye health. Toxic to cancer cells
Iodine	Aim for 3 drops of Lugol's 15% at night	Clean up the upper fermenting gut	Essential for antioxidant status (to neutralise free radicals). Contact kills all microbes. Anti-inflammatory and anti-allergic. Binds to toxic metals to help excretion. Essential to make thyroid hormones, sex hormones and oxytocin (the love hormone)
Vitamin B12	5 mg methyl B12 in Sunshine Salt B12 injections ½ ml x 1 mg/ml daily Trial for 2 months – if better, then use as often as is needed to maintain benefits	Great for the foggy brain 'The only way you could kill yourself with B12 is to drown in the stuff' says Dr Chris Dawkins, environmental physician (and good friend)	Probably by improving mitochondrial function. Relieves depression. Anti-inflammatory – mops up the pro-inflammatory peroxynitrite and nitric oxide. Essential for the methylation cycle – protein synthesis ergo healing, repair and detoxing. Directly toxic to some viruses (e.g. hepatitis C). Often relieves restless legs

Tools	Dose	Their primary job	What they also do
Heating regimes	At least weekly sunshine, sauna-ing, farinfrared sauna-ing and/ or…	Eliminates through the skin all volatile organic compounds and pesticides	See Chapter 14 on how to reduce the toxic burden
Epsom salt baths	At least weekly	Eliminates through the skin all volatile organic compounds and pesticides	Also delivers a good dose of magnesium (for mitochondrial function and muscle relaxation and more) and sulphate (for detoxing and to improve the fourth phase of water[7])
DMSO	Aim for 20 ml daily	Improves the fourth phase water[7] and therefore blood and lymphatic circulation	Essential raw material for connective tissue – reduces the friction, so great for tendonitis, bursitis, capsulitis. Use with magnesium transdermally and topically for any of the above. Antioxidant. Anti-inflammatory and analgesic

It is time to lighten the load a little with a couple of jokes about mitochondria – yes these exist!

Q: What's the difference between mitochondria and a home's solar panels?
A: One is the powerhouse of the cell; the other is the power cell of the house.

Q/A: Did you know that, according to scientists, in October the mitochondria turn into the frightochondria?
And become the haunted house of the cell.

But best of all is the internet meme on page 216, which really does sum up this chapter in one.

Summary

- Our first published paper showed that among my CFS patients those with the worst levels of fatigue had the worst mitochondrial function.
- Our third published paper showed that tailored regimes of supplements and other interventions, such as detoxing, improved mitochondrial function.
- We have a 'Mitochondrial Package' of supplements, detox regimes, pacing and avoidance of toxic load that improve mitochondrial function and should be taken by all CFS sufferers.
- There is no need to test your mitochondrial function – just do the package as above.

Chapter 6

Oxygen

Oxygen – even I know what happens when my cylinder runs out!

Coal miner with pneumoconiosis, Annesley Woodhouse, Nottinghamshire circa 1985*

For mitochondria to 'burn' fuel efficiently (aerobically), they need oxygen. Intuitively one might think that to get more oxygen to our mitochondria we need to breathe more and take deep breaths. Wrong! This has the opposite effect. To get oxygen to our mitochondria we must breathe less. Why so?

The science†

Our lungs are not primarily designed to acquire oxygen; they evolved to hang on to carbon dioxide (CO_2). CO_2 dissolves in plasma as carbonic acid and this controls when and where red blood cells, containing the oxygen-carrying molecule haemoglobin, either grab or release oxygen. In the lungs, CO_2 levels are low so oxygen sticks to

***Footnote:** Craig's beloved Scully,† of *The X Files*, made a similar comment in Season 1, Episode 8.

†**Footnote:** 'The Scully Effect' – Gillian Anderson played the role of Special Agent Dana Scully and, as fans will know, was the logical 'scientific' lead, whereas Special Agent Fox Mulder (played by David Duchovny) was the 'believer' of all things paranormal and alien. So powerful was the role of Scully that it led to 'The Scully Effect', a phenomenon whereby the number of women starting careers in typical STEM (science/technology/engineering/mathematics) professions saw a noticeable increase following the airing of the *X-Files* in the early 1990s. This Effect was confirmed by a study carried out by the Geena Davis Institute on Gender in Media.[1]

haemoglobin. In the tissues where CO_2 is the exhaust gas of busy mitochondria, CO_2 levels are high and so oxygen is released from haemoglobin. The mechanism is acidity: with low carbonic acid in the lungs, oxygen is grabbed; with high carbonic acid in the tissues, oxygen is released.

This does make good physiological sense. It means that oxygen is delivered precisely to working mitochondria and not wasted where it is not needed. To do otherwise would be horribly inefficient. I shall be boring and repeat these points because this is such an important concept:

> Lungs – low CO_2, alkali blood, oxygen sticks to haemoglobin.
>
> Mitochondria – high CO_2, acid blood, oxygen is released from haemoglobin.

The effects of over-breathing

Many people, for many reasons, over-breathe. Often this is driven by the stress hormone adrenalin. This has the disastrous metabolic effect of washing CO_2 out of the bloodstream. Blood becomes too alkali and oxygen sticks more avidly to haemoglobin… and remains stuck there! This means that oxygen delivery to our mitochondria is impaired. Instead of oxygen being released it remains trapped in haemoglobin. Mitochondria are starved of oxygen and symptoms result.

Table 6.1: The what, why and how of over-breathing

What – the symptoms	Why	How to treat
Obviously, fatigue. All the symptoms of poor energy delivery to the body, the brain and the heart (see Chapter 2)	If you cannot get oxygen to your mitochondria, then they will go slow	Do the breathing exercises below

What – the symptoms	Why	How to treat
Mouth-breathing	This reduces the dead space of respiration. Less exhaled air is re-inhaled and so more CO_2 is expelled. The 'dead space' is the volume of air that remains in the airways with exhalation. Relative to air it is rich in CO_2. This is re-inhaled and helps to maintain the acidity of the blood	NEVER breathe through your mouth. Even with exercise. Many athletes improve their performance by nasal breathing. Mouth breathing is only necessary with extreme demands when mitochondria are producing huge amounts of CO_2
...which results in dry mouth	The nose has a delicate system of turbinates to warm and moisturise air that is inhaled. Mouth-breathers lose much water	Shut your mouth!
Tooth decay and gum disease	Microbes in the mouth love oxygen	Nose-breathe And of course, avoid carbs in the diet
Long-term mouth-breathing changes the anatomy. resulting in nasal obstruction, crowded teeth and undershot jaw	The pressures within the upper airways pull and push the airways into shape. The more you nose-breathe the more open the passages become	Shut your mouth! When talking, learn to breathe in through your nose and then speak
Sinusitis	Mouth-breathing means the sinuses are not aerated and so prone to infection. Mucus in the nose is not properly circulated. The more you mouth-breathe the more the nasal cavities collapse	Open up the nasal airways by sniffing iodine with a salt pipe or sniffing essential oils such as wintergreen. Then keep them open with nasal breathing. If you do not use it you lose it!
		Do breathing exercises, one nostril at a time (see below)
Snoring and sleep apnoea	The upper airways are not inflated, become narrow and collapse during sleep	Nose-breathe Tape your mouth shut at night

Table 6.1 *Cont'd*

What – the symptoms	Why	How to treat
Asthma…	The bronchoconstriction of asthma is an attempt by the body to retain CO_2. Unfortunately, it has the opposite effect – the brain panics and produces adrenalin which drives respiration	Asthma can be reversed with the breathing exercises below. You can reduce the adrenalin with slow breathing and diaphragmatic breathing
…and chronic obstructive airways disease (COPD)	Mucus build-up in the lungs is again an attempt by the body to retain CO_2	COPD can be greatly improved by the exercises below. Avoid dairy products, which produce catarrh. Sniff iodine in a salt pipe to deal with any infection. Iodine is also anti-allergic
Autonomic nervous system imbalance – Too much sympathetic drive resulting in fight-or-flight and causing high blood pressure, tachycardia, anxiety, diarrhoea, perhaps tremor, sweating and insomnia	If the brain perceives that it is not getting oxygen to its mitochondria, then it panics and generates adrenalin. This drives hyperventilation and makes things much worse – a real vicious cycle	Do the breathing exercises below
Too little parasympathetic action (associated with 'rest and digest') leading to poor gut function: indigestion, bloating, constipation	With hyperventilation, breathing takes place with the chest muscles instead of the diaphragm. The diaphragm does at least two important jobs: not only does it suck air in from the nose, but the negative pressure generated also sucks blood into the chest for the rest of the body, thereby improving circulation	Learn diaphragmatic breathing
	The diaphragm massages the whole of the gut, liver, pancreas, spleen and kidneys and stimulates blood and lymphatic circulation	Learn diaphragmatic breathing

What – the symptoms	Why	How to treat
Shortness of breath is a feature of long Covid – almost certainly this is hyperventilation	The mechanism of this is not clear. Possibly infection of the vagus nerve, possibly the pro-inflammatory effect of spike protein	Do the breathing exercises below

Please note that a pulse oximeter measures the oxygen saturation of haemoglobin. It does not reflect oxygen delivery to the tissues. Just because you may have good oxygen saturation does *not* mean that there is good oxygen delivery to your tissues.[2]

How to prevent over-breathing

In summary: (1) nose-breathe, (2) learn to use your diaphragm , (3) slow your breathing down.

1. *First* learn to nose-breathe:
   - To begin you need to open up your nostrils. Cut out dairy products, which are catarrh forming. Breathing through the nostrils should be silent – any noise suggests blockage. Clear this by sniffing iodine. Put 2 drops of 15% Lugol's iodine into the mouthpiece of a salt pipe and sniff this. You should be able to smell the iodine. Often this mobilises mucus, which you can clear by 'hawking' it to the back of your throat, so it can be swallowed. Essential oils are often effective, such as eucalyptus or wintergreen.
   - Test one nostril at a time by closing off one with your thumb. If blocked, then sniff iodine or oils through the blockage. You should be able to breathe noiselessly at rest through one nostril.
   - Once the nasal passages are clear, keep them so by never mouth-breathing. Keep your mouth shut!
2. *Then* breathe with your diaphragm:
   - The body can suck air into the lungs in two ways – with the diaphragm and with the chest muscles. At rest we should largely use the diaphragm for all the reasons detailed above. When physical demands are high, such as when we are sprinting at the end of a long hunt in order to catch our prey, the chest muscles are additionally employed, but this should be a rare event when adrenalin is running high.

- When you use your diaphragm to breathe, your tummy should rise and fall with each breath and your chest remain still.
- To learn to do this, lie down and put your right hand over your tummy button and the left over your heart. Breathe so only your right hand moves and the left stays still. Once you get the idea, you can do this walking around, sitting or whatever.

3. NOW YOU ARE READY to slow your breathing down:
    - We should breathe between five and six diaphragmatic breaths per minute with normal activity. At rest, do the exercises below to slow this even further to reset the respiratory rate.
    - Lie or sit down at rest with a watch that has a second hand.
    - Start with a full cycle every 10 seconds. Breathe in slowly for 4 seconds, then out for 4 seconds, then hold for 2 seconds. Use the muscles at the back of your nose to slightly constrict the exit of air through your nose and increase the pressure in your airways. This should feel very comfortable. Do this for 2 minutes.
    - Then extend the cycle to every 12 seconds. Breathe in slowly for 4 seconds, out for 5 seconds then hold for 3 seconds. Do this for 2 minutes.
    - Extend the cycle to every 15 seconds. Breathe in slowly for 4 seconds, out for 6 seconds and really squeeze out every last bit of air from your lungs.
    - Keep extending the cycle until you start to get 'air hunger' – that is to say, you have an over-whelming need to take a deep breath. Resist this. Now you are resetting your breathing 'thermostat'; you are retraining your respiratory centre in the brain not to panic.
    - It should be very possible to get down to three breaths per minute at rest. There may be a mild sensation of air hunger. Resist the urge to gasp. You will be massively improving your oxygen delivery to your mitochondria.

Diaphragmatic breathing

The diaphragm is not only responsible for breathing; it is also essential for returning venous blood to the heart:

- As we breathe in, the diaphragm descends, and this sucks venous blood into the chest and squeezes venous blood from the abdomen up into the chest.
- As we breathe out, the diaphragm ascends, and sucks venous blood into the abdomen from the legs.

- Ditto in the lungs – inhalation draws blood into the lungs from the heart and exhalation squeezes the blood from the lungs back to the heart.

Other things you can do to retrain your breathing

Other ways to retrain your breathing include:

- Singing – This involves long exhalations. That is good.
- Humming through your nose. Apparently I can't sing. I think I can, but my girls tell me I can't. So it is not a good option for me.
- Learn to play a wind instrument – Again this involves long exhalations.
- When you talk, make a conscious effort to breathe in through your nose. I know some people who can start a sentence before they have finished the one before! They are mouth-breathers.
- When you go walking or jogging, keep you mouth shut. Again, there may be an early sensation of air hunger and a desire to open your mouth and gasp. Resist it! Emil Zátopek[‡] won four Olympic gold medals and broke 18 world records running with under-ventilation training. He did all the above. Even for him it was painful resisting the air hunger, but it worked. He had more energy.
- When you go walking, exhale, hold your breath and keep walking, count your steps until air hunger makes you want to breathe again. Aim to increase the number of steps.

[‡]**Historical note:** Emil Zátopek (19 September 1922 – 21 November 2000) was a Czech long-distance runner. He won a gold medal in the 10,000 metres at the London Olympics of 1948, a race witnessed by Craig's father, and then three gold medals at the 1952 Summer Olympics in Helsinki. At that meet, he won gold in the 5000 metres and 10,000 metres runs, but his final medal came when he decided at the last minute to compete in the first marathon of his life. His wife, Dana Zátopková (born the same day and year as Emil), won a gold medal in the javelin at the 1952 Olympics, only a few moments after Emil's victory in the 5000 metres. Emil playfully attempted to take some credit for his wife's Olympic victory at her press conference, claiming that it was his victory in the 5000 metres that had 'inspired' her. Dana's response was perfect: 'Really? Okay, go inspire some other girl and see if she throws a javelin 50 metres!'

Wim Hof breathing

Wim Hof breathing is another technique for re-training your breathing.

Wim Hof (born 20 April 1959), also known as the 'Iceman', is a Dutch motivational speaker and extreme athlete, noted for his ability to withstand low temperatures. He holds the Guinness record for a barefoot half marathon on ice and snow.

We should not lead lives that are too comfortable, and it is a good idea to shake things up occasionally. Wim Hof has demonstrated great benefits from episodes of forced hyperventilation – that is, over-breathing. Only do this lying down until you become familiar with the symptoms generated. Breathe in as deeply as you can for 3 seconds then out for 3 seconds and really squeeze all the air out. Keep going for 30 breaths. This process takes 3 minutes. At your last exhalation, stop with your lungs not squeezed out but relaxed and hold your breath. Many find they do not need to breathe for 2 or 3 minutes! Hold your breath until air hunger prevails. Repeat for three cycles.

One should be left with a feeling of peace and calmness. I believe this is medicated by endorphins. In this brief window of hyperventilation, we are mimicking the breathing patten that comes with a great excitement, such as hunting our prey or having sex, and that too is followed by a pulse of endorphins.

Summary

- Mitochondria need oxygen.
- To get oxygen into our mitochondria we must breathe *less*.
- Over-breathing causes many problems including:
  - Fatigue
  - Tooth decay and gum disease
  - Crowded teeth, undershot jaw
  - Sinusitis
  - Sleep apnoea

  - Asthma
  - Chronic obstructive airways disease (COPD)
  - Autonomic nervous system imbalance
    - Too much sympathetic drive
    - Too little parasympathetic action
- Address over-breathing by:
  - Nose-breathing
  - Breathing using your diaphragm
  - Practising slowing your breathing down
  - Using other techniques such as
    - Singing
    - Humming through your nose
    - Learning to play a wind instrument
    - Trying Wim Hof breathing
- In summary, KEEP YOUR MOUTH SHUT!

Chapter 7

The thyroid accelerator pedal and the adrenal gear box

We sort of just took up by the river one day, we don't belong to each other: he's an independent and, so am I.

Holly speaking in *Breakfast at Tiffany's*,* the novella, by Truman Garcia Capote (1924 – 1984), American novelist, screenwriter, playwright and actor

In quoting this line, what is my point? It is that, though the thyroid and adrenals *can* be treated separately, often one finds that they will need simultaneous treatment, and so, although they don't 'belong to each other', they do 'live' next door to each other. (Metaphorically, not actually!).This is why they are dealt with in the same chapter. And, to use the car analogy (see Chapter 2), how can one use the gearbox without the accelerator pedal and vice versa? Again, this chapter is written on the need-to-know basis – much more information can be found in our book *The Underactive Thyroid: Do it yourself because your doctor won't.*

The rate at which our mitochondrial engines go is controlled by thyroid hormones which give us an average speed, and this is then fine-tuned by adrenal hormones which closely match energy supply to energy demands. Adrenalin increases energy delivery in seconds to minutes, cortisol in minutes to hours and DHEA in hours to days. Adrenal and thyroid

***Literary aside from Craig:** Sarah bought me a year's subscription to Audible for my birthday and this was the first book I listened to. So much better than the (excellent) film with Audrey Hepburn.

fatigues are common. The underactive adrenal gland is never diagnosed by doctors and the underactive thyroid is under-diagnosed and under-treated. This is because doctors rely entirely on blood tests to diagnose and monitor patients and completely ignore the clinical picture, symptoms and signs. What this means is – as our sub-title says – that you have to do it yourself because your doctor won't.

If your energy levels are not improving on the PK diet (page 22), vitamin C and iodine, the Basic Package of supplements (page 43) and the mitochondrial package (page 54), then the thyroid and adrenals are your next port of call.

The history, symptoms and signs of the underactive thyroid

Be suspicious with any or all of the symptoms of poor energy delivery mechanisms described in Chapter 5. In addition, we have the symptoms and signs listed in Table 7.1.

Table 7.1: Symptoms of the underactive thyroid and mechanisms that underlie them

Mechanism	Symptom	Notes
Fluid retention and oedema	Puffy face	Compare current looks with old photographs
	Large tongue	You may see indentations from where teeth lie against the tongue
	Obstructive sleep apnoea perhaps with snoring	Because the tissues of the throat are swollen, and this constricts the airways
	Voice changes	The vocal cords are puffy
	Swollen, puffy legs, most obvious in the ankles at the end of the day	A cause of 'non-pitting' oedema
	Nerves get squashed e.g. carpal tunnel syndrome, sciatica	
Poor fat burning	Ketogenic hypoglycaemia: On a PK diet you need thyroid hormones to burn fat – if low, then fat burning is done with adrenalin, and this gives all the symptoms of low blood sugar	The symptoms of low blood sugar are not due to low blood sugar but the adrenalin (and other hormonal) responses to low blood sugar

Table 7.1 *Cont'd*

Mechanism	Symptom	Notes
Sleep disturbance	Poor quality unrefreshing sleep	
	This is well recognised in hypothyroidism but the mechanism is uncertain. It may in part be due to sleep disturbance by ketogenic hypoglycaemia	
	Being an owl (drop off to sleep late, wake late) and so feeling 'jet-lagged'	There are at least three groups of hormones for quality sleep and correct diurnal rhythm. Light inhibits melatonin production while dark stimulates such. Melatonin stimulates the pituitary and so TSH spikes at midnight. Then T4 spikes at 4 am and T3 at 5 am and this stimulates the production of adrenal hormones which wake us up
Proximal myopathy – i.e. symmetrical weakness of proximal upper and/or lower limbs (thigh and/or upper arm)	May present with difficulty climbing hills or stairs, trouble getting out of the bath or off the floor or even up from a chair. Or getting on to a horse! Press-ups become impossible	Often misdiagnosed as lack of fitness
I am not sure of the mechanism of this – probably a combination of poor energy delivery and being cold together with oedema of the gut	Constipation	Constipation is often an early symptom to improve once the underactive thyroid has been corrected
Again, I am not sure of the mechanism of this	Headaches	Clinically, headaches often settle with thyroid glandulars

Table 7.2: Signs of the underactive thyroid – useful for diagnosing and monitoring

Sign	Mechanism	Notes
Low core temperature – e.g. below 36.8°C[†]	Poor energy delivery	Monitoring core temperature is helpful to get the dose of thyroid and adrenal supplements right
Low blood pressure – e.g. below 110/70 mm Hg	Poor energy delivery to the heart so it cannot beat powerfully	This may well be masked by the adrenalin of metabolic syndrome (a pre-diabetic condition) or ketogenic hypoglycaemia
Slow pulse – i.e. less than 70 beats per minute (bpm) in a non-athlete	The thyroid is largely responsible for the resting pulse rate	A normal person, not in athletic training should have a resting pulse of 70-75 bpm Again, this may be masked by adrenalin as above

[†]**Footnote from Craig:** 'C' for 'Centigrade' or for 'Celsius'? Centigrade, we are told, is an historical forerunner to the Celsius temperature scale. Centigrade is from the Latin *centum*, which means 100, and *gradus*, which means steps, and so there are 100 equal divisions (steps) between the freezing point and boiling water of water, in the Centigrade scale. The Celsiuis scale is exactly the same as the Centigrade scale. It is named after the Swedish astronomer Anders Celsius (1701–1744), who developed a variant of it in 1742. Most countries use the Celsius scale; the other major scale, Fahrenheit, is still used in the United States, some island territories, and Liberia. Daily newspapers in the UK seem to use Fahrenheit when the temperature is hot, because they can report high numbers (e.g. 80ºF, which would seem far cooler if expressed in Celsius, at around 26ºC) and use Celsius when the temperature is cold because they can report low numbers then (e.g. -7ºC, which would look far warmer if expressed in Fahrenheit – around 19ºF). For me, the most famous temperature in Fahrenheit is 451, the supposed burning temperature of books in the classic book by Ray Bradbury, *Fahrenheit 451* about a dystopian future where firefighters burn books rather than put out fires, and much more. Both Sarah and I are glad that such firefighters do not exist in this world, so that our books can be read and enjoyed by so many of you, without fear of a knock on the door from your local 'firefighter'!
The formula connecting Fahrenheit and Celsius is:

$F = {}^{\circ}C \times 1.8 + 32$

So, given a temperature in Celsius multiply that by 1.8 and then add 32 to get the temperature in Fahrenheit. It follows that the only temperature at which Fahrenheit and Celsius agree is -40, and so -40ºF = -40ºC. (That's enough, Craig. Stop! Sarah)

Medical history of the underactive thyroid

Table 7.3: Medical history – useful for suspecting the diagnosis

What	Why	Notes
Being female	Taking the Pill and HRT are both major risk factors for the underactive thyroid	Women with CFS/ME outnumber men by at least 4:1.[1] Baha Arafah concluded women who were receiving oestrogen therapy, and who were also hypothyroid, had an increased need for thyroxine[2]
Family history	Thyroid problems run in families, especially down the female line	Possibly genetic[3] but families have the same diet and environmental and infectious exposures. Genetics does not mean that there is nothing that can be done!
Other autoimmune conditions	Autoimmunity runs in families[3]	Again, possibly genetic. Again, families have the same diet and environmental and infectious exposures
Gradual decline into ill health	The thyroid may be slowly destroyed by autoimmunity, micronutrient deficiency, toxins, radiation…	All the above symptoms are ascribed by doctors to age, stress, menopause etcetera, so patients are dismissed without proper clinical consideration. This is further reason to do it yourself
	…and prescription medications: lithium,[4] amiodarone,[5] beta blockers[6]	But probably many others
Triggers:		
1. vaccines	These are good at triggering autoimmune disease. Covid mRNA gene therapy 'vaccines' are no exception	Not wishing to 'clutter' this book, interested readers can see our book *The Underactive Thyroid* for a list of 31 studies supporting the fact that vaccines trigger autoimmune diseases. See also, as an example only:, 'Two Cases of Graves' Disease Following SARS-CoV-2 Vaccination: An Autoimmune/Inflammatory Syndrome Induced by Adjuvants'[7]

What	Why	Notes
2. menopause	Progesterone increases the efficacy of thyroid hormones	The menopause and its associated fall in progesterone may unmask underlying hypothyroidism
		In consequence many women have been wrongly prescribed progesterone (when the underactive thyroid diagnosis has been missed) and this is dangerous medicine: progesterone is carcinogenic
3. viral infection	May present with an overactive thyroid and this progresses to an underactive thyroid, typically women aged 40-50 triggered in summer and early autumn	So-called sub-acute thyroiditis (SAT) – e.g. there is evidence of SAT being preceded by upper respiratory tract infection, and of elevated viral antibody levels, and both seasonal and geographical clustering of cases[8]
4. whiplash	A good friend and osteopath has noticed this association	This is biologically plausible as there may well be soft tissue injury. I reckon my underactive thyroid dates from three broken necks (sigh, yes – that is horses for you!)

All diagnosis is hypothesis which we then put to the test by treating and seeing the response. If your clinical picture fits the bill, then firstly one needs to do blood tests, not so much to diagnose the underactive thyroid as to make sure you are not overactive, though this is rare.

One can be underactive for many possible reasons vis:

- The thyroid gland has failed.
- The pituitary gland has failed.
- You are not converting inactive T4 to the active form, T3.
- You have high levels of reverse T3 (which blocks active T3).
- You have thyroid hormone receptor resistance.

Regardless of the mechanism, the treatment is the same – a trial of thyroid glandulars (TGs). The key to this is to start with a low dose, increase very slowly and monitor by how you feel (all the symptoms above), pulse rate at rest and core temperature. There is a 'sweet spot'. It is easy to overshoot this because thyroid hormones are long-acting with the potential to bioaccumulate *and* they determine the number of mitochondria within cells (the size of your 'engine').

- Start with thyroid glandular 15 mg sublingually on rising.
- After one week take a second capsule midday (this is because the active T3 is shorter acting so you can be fired up for the morning and again for the afternoon).
- Increase in 15-mg increments every week.

The eventual dose is partly weight dependent. Most people need TGs 60 mg porcine (TGs 65 mg bovine) which is 1-3 capsules daily depending on body weight.

A typical dose would be:

- up to 9 stone (57 kg) – 1-2 capsules daily (i.e. porcine glandular 60-120 mg)
- up to 12 stone (76 kg) – 1-3 capsules daily (i.e. porcine glandular 60-180 mg)
- up to 15 stone (95 kg) – 2-4 capsules daily (i.e. porcine glandular 120-240 mg)
- Above 15 stone (+95 kg) – 2-5 capsules daily (i.e. porcine glandular 120-300 mg)

For those used to 'old money', 60 mg of porcine TG (65 mg of bovine TG) is equivalent to one grain of armour thyroid. See the Useful Resources section for details of suppliers of these supplements and glandulars (page 303).

The adrenal gearbox

The symptoms and signs of the underactive adrenal gland are not as clear as those of the underactive thyroid. Neither is the treatment. It is largely a case of clinical suspicion followed by trial and error. An adrenal saliva stress test is often useful. Medichecks can provide the adrenal saliva stress test (see page 308).

The history, symptoms and signs of underactive adrenal glands

Again, any or all of the symptoms of poor energy delivery mechanisms (see Chapter 5) are relevant. Then, a history of unremitting stress plus the symptoms listed in Table 7.4.

Unremitting stress is a very important clue. This often starts in childhood with sexual, physical, mental or emotional abuse. It may date from a terrifying experience with post-traumatic stress. Either way, the victim becomes hypervigilant and runs their life on adrenalin, often turning to addiction (sugar, nicotine, alcohol, prescription drugs etc) to relieve those ghastly symptoms. All this exhausts the adrenals. Simply correcting the adrenal dysfunction will not reverse past horrors, but it will give energy and possibly sleep to allow psychological tools to be more effective.

Table 7.4: The symptoms of underactive adrenal glands and their underlying mechanisms

Mechanism	Symptom	Notes
Adrenal hormones allow us to gear up to stress by increasing energy delivery	Stress intolerance – an inability to rise to the occasion to deal with the unexpected	Stress is an essential part of life. Modest stress makes us stronger. Excessive, unremitting stress shortens life.
Adrenal hormones should be highest in the morning and decline through the day	Coming to life during the late afternoon or evening. Being an owl – drop off to sleep late, wake late	
As adrenal glands fatigue, those hormone levels that we measure clinically drop in a particular order – first sex hormones…	Loss of libido	Do not try to correct this with sex hormones. These give false energy. Oestrogen and progesterone are a major risk for cancer (growth promoting) and heart disease (pro-inflammatory)
…then DHEA, followed by cortisol and finally adrenalin. Normally the stimulating effects of adrenalin are mitigated by cortisol and DHEA	Feel wired but tired with inability to drop off to sleep, poor quality sleep and exaggerated startle reflex	

Table 7.4 *Cont'd*

Mechanism	Symptom	Notes
Adrenal hormones control inflammation in the body	With adrenal fatigue there is a tendency to inflammatory conditions such as allergy and autoimmunity together with an increased susceptibility to infection	
Control of salt and water balance via mineralocorticoids (steroid hormones that regulate salt and water balance)	Craving for salt, tendency to dehydration, possibly frequent micturition (need to pee), tendency to low blood pressure, muscle cramps	
Adrenal hormones are partly responsible for core temperature	Wobbly core temperature – if this varies by much more than 0.6°C this may point to adrenal fatigue	Wobbly core temperature may also point to a chronic infection – fever kills microbes – and may represent a poor attempt to do such
Adrenalin is cleared in the blood by catechol-O-methyltransferases	It is biologically plausible that high adrenalin symptoms may be due to poor methylation	Check homocysteine (a marker of poor methylation). This can be reduced with methyl vitamin B12 5 mg, methyl-tetrahydro folic acid 800 mcg and pyridoxal-5-phosphate 50 mg

Adrenal stress test (saliva)

The adrenal stress test (ASP) measures levels of cortisol, DHEA (and melatonin on request) over 24 hours. This is the most useful test because salivary levels of DHEA and cortisol are accurate (arguably better than blood tests because blood tests are skewed by protein binding and the stress of undergoing blood testing), the tests can be done in the less stressful environment at home and are easily available to all (see Useful resources, page 303).

Normally one expects to see high levels of cortisol and DHEA in the morning which fall as the day progresses. The level of DHEA should be commensurate with the cortisol.

Patterns of abnormality are as shown in Table 7.5.

Table 7.5: Interpretation of an ASP

Significant result	What it means	Action
Cortisol and/or DHEA spikes above the upper limit at any time of day	Indicates a stress response as DHEA follows cortisol which follows adrenalin	Identify the cause of the stress. The commonest cause is the falling blood sugar of metabolic syndrome in the patient who is not keto-adapted – i.e. do the PK diet
	The adrenal gland is working okay but it, and the whole body, is stressed. This is not sustainable long term, and a crash is on the horizon	Again, identify the cause of the stress. Look for ways to reduce the demands on your life – physical, mental, emotional, financial, social, infectious and so on
Low DHEA, normal cortisol	The adrenal gland is starting to fatigue	Ditto above. Start adrenal support as below
Very low DHEA, low cortisol	More of the above	Ditto
	Adrenalin is the last hormone to go down; high levels are not mitigated by cortisol and DHEA ergo 'wired but tired'	
	Poor quality sleep	Ditto above. Consider melatonin 3-9 mg at night. Take sublingually
Flattening of the circadian rhythm	Points to hypothyroidism	Sort out the thyroid
	All the above are accompanied by falling levels of sex hormones with loss of libido. This is Nature telling you that you do not have the reserves and energy for procreation	Do not suppress symptoms with HRT – this is dangerous medicine. HRT is growth promoting (risk for cancer), immunosuppressive (risk of infection) and pro-thrombotic (risk for heart attack and stroke). I never bother to measure sex hormones as this does not change management

Treatment of adrenal fatigue

There are two essential steps: to take the pressure off and feed the adrenals, and then to reduce their workload with herbals and glandulars.

1. Take the pressure off the adrenals and feed them

In summary, what we are looking at here is:

- Reducing demands through pacing and reducing addictions.
- Restoring with sleep and rest.
- Providing the right ingredients for recovery with Groundhog Basic (see Appendix 1).

Essentially, the adrenals become fatigued because the body does not have the energy to deal with the demands it faces. In the short term, much can be achieved on adrenalin, but this is not sustainable in the long term. Look for ways to reduce the demands on your life – nutritional, physical, mental, emotional, financial, social etc. This is called pacing – it is very boring but the better you pace the quicker will be your recovery.

Note that addictions are stressful and addressing these will reduce stress. They include: carbohydrates, caffeine, alcohol, nicotine.

The adrenal glands restore with rest so it is worth working to get good sleep (see Chapter 8) and try: naps in the day, meditation, taking weekends off and allowing yourself holidays.

The adrenals are particularly demanding of vitamin B5, vitamin C, salt and fats. These are all part of Groundhog Basic (Appendix 1). We need fat for cholesterol, which is the starting point to synthesise all glucocorticoids, mineralocorticoids and sex hormones.

2. Reduce the work of the adrenals with herbals and adrenal glandulars

There are no hard and fast rules here and it really is a case of trial and error. The most useful to try, possibly in combination, are:

- Ashwagandha – start with 1 gram (g); some people take up to 4 g daily.
- Ginseng – use 1-3 g of the root powder.
- Bovine adrenal glandular – cortex 150-450 mg.
- Pregnenolone 25-100 mg – this is the most upstream of the adrenal hormones, also dubbed the memory hormone.
- DHEA 25-100 mg.

The use of any of the above in these doses does not suppress adrenal function. The idea is to plug a gap where such exists – to prop up and support whilst the adrenal glands recover. This renders these treatments extremely safe. By contrast, mainstream doctors prescribe adrenal hormones in huge, non-physiological, immune-suppressing doses which switch off endogenous production and cause long-term life-threatening side effects. The commonest steroid used is prednisolone (*not* to be confused with pregnenolone). Even the dose of steroids in asthma inhaler medications, nasal sprays and skin creams may be sufficient to cause adrenal suppression.

Final general advice

If you have symptoms of salt and water balance problems, start by increasing salt and fat in your diet, then add in liquorice (1-5 g root powder – *not* the sweet, black stuff otherwise known as 'All Sorts').

Finally, all such hormones (thyroid, adrenal, melatonin) are best taken sublingually (under the tongue). They get straight into the bloodstream via the mouth. Swallowed and the first port of call is the liver, which detoxes them. Some get through but you get more bang for your buck taking them sublingually.

See the Useful Resources section (page 303) for details of suppliers of these supplements and glandulars.

Summary

- If all is in place from Chapters 4-6, and Chapters 8 and 9, and there is little improvement, then look at the thyroid and adrenal glands.
- Often the thyroid and adrenals need to be treated together.
- Use medical history, symptoms and signs to diagnose an underactive thyroid and treat with thyroid glandulars. (For more detail see our book *The Underactive Thyroid*.)
- Use the adrenal stress profile (saliva test) to diagnose adrenal problems and treat with:
    - 'Taking the pressure off'
    - Groundhog Basic
    - Herbals
    - Glandulars
    - Pregnenolone
    - DHEA.

Chapter 8

Sleep – when healing and repair take place

Sleep is the golden chain that ties health and our bodies together.

Thomas Dekker (c.1572 – 1632)

Why we sleep

All living creatures have times in their cycle when they shut down their metabolic activity for healing and repair to take place. In higher animals we call this sleep. During the 'flu epidemic after the First World War, a few sufferers developed neurological damage in which they lost the ability to sleep. All were dead within two weeks; this was the first solid evidence that sleep is an absolute essential for life.* Happily, the body has a symptom which tells us how much sleep we need. It is called tiredness – ignore this at your peril. During sleep we heal and repair; during our waking hours we cause cell damage. If there is insufficient sleep, then the cell damage exceeds healing and repair, and our health gradually ratchets downhill. Lack of sleep is a major risk factor for all

*__A salutary lesson:__ Why would he do it, but in December 1963/January 1964, 17-year-old Randy Gardner stayed awake for 11 days and 24 minutes (264.4 hours) in order to break the Guinness world record. Lt Cmdr John J Ross monitored his cognitive and behavioural health and reported serious complications. These included moodiness, problems with concentration and short-term memory loss, paranoia and hallucinations. On the 11th day, when Gardner was asked to subtract seven repeatedly, starting with 100, he stopped at 65. When asked why he had stopped, he replied that he had forgotten what he was doing. Decades later, Gardner reported still suffering from occasional, but worrying, cognitive symptoms and also serious insomnia.

degenerative conditions from heart disease to cancer and neurological disorders.

During sleep the glymphatics, the rubbish disposal systems of the brain, open up to allow cleaning, healing and repair. An example of the 'rubbish' they clean up is amyloid, the pathological protein of Alzheimer's disease. This is cleared from the brain during sleep. If sleep is lacking, then amyloid builds up. Lack of sleep is a, possibly *the*, major risk factor for dementia. Indeed, there is no disease process that is not worsened by lack of sleep. It really is a risk factor for all disease. Quantity and quality of sleep are non-negotiable. Without a good night's sleep on a regular basis, all other interventions are to no avail.

There are at least three aspects to pay attention to: the quantity of sleep, when to sleep (circadian rhythm) and the quality of sleep.

The quantity of sleep

Modern Western man is chronically sleep deprived. He averages 7.5 hours' sleep when the biological average requirement is nearer 9 hours, perhaps a bit more in winter, less in summer. To show how critical this balance is, imagine dividing the day into 12 hours of activity and 12 hours of rest. One extra hour of damaging activity (13 hours) means the loss of one hour of rest and healing sleep (11 hours). The difference is 2 hours. It is vital to observe a regular bedtime and be able to wake naturally, without an alarm clock, feeling refreshed.

When to sleep (circadian† rhythm)

Humans evolved to sleep when it is dark and wake when it is light. Sleep is a form of hibernation when the body shuts down in order to repair damage done through use, to conserve energy and to hide from predators. The normal sleep pattern that evolved

†**Historical note:** Franz Halberg (5 July 1919 – 9 June 2013) coined the word 'circadian' in 1959 by combining two Latin words: *circa* (about) and *diem*, accusative singular of *dies* (day). Halberg was a maverick, working seven days a week, right up to his death, who spoke of the 'quicksand of clinical trials on groups' and that 'These [clinical trials] ignore individual differences and hence the individual's needs.'[1]

in hot climates is to sleep, keep warm and conserve energy during the cold nights and then sleep again in the afternoons when it is too hot to work, and to hide away from the midday sun. As humans migrated away from the Equator, the sleep pattern had to change with the seasons and as the lengths of the days changed. In winter we need to shut down to conserve energy; this means more sleep. Mild fatigue and depression prevent us from spending energy unnecessarily. Conversely, in the summer we need to expend large amounts of energy to harvest the summer bounties and accumulate reserves to carry us through the winter; we naturally need less sleep, can work longer hours and have more energy. But the need for a rest (if not a sleep) in the middle of the day is still there. Therefore, it is no surprise that young children, the elderly and people who become ill often have an extra sleep in the afternoon, and for these people that is totally desirable. Others have learned to 'power nap', as it is called, during the day and this allows them to feel more energetic later. If you can do it, then this is an excellent habit to get into; it can be learned.

My father was a napper, he called it his 'short course of death' – Sarah

The average daily sleep requirement is 9 hours, ideally taken between 9.30 pm and 6.30 am – that is, during the hours of darkness – but allow for more in the winter and less in the summer. An hour of sleep before midnight is worth two after; this is because human growth hormone is produced during the hours of sleep before midnight.

The symptom of jet lag is a powerful illustration of the existence of a circadian rhythm. This starts with light which impacts on the skin (interestingly not necessarily through the eyes) and switches off the production of melatonin, the body's natural sleep hormone. As darkness ensues, melatonin is produced to create the hormonal environment for sleep. Melatonin stimulates the pituitary gland to produce thyroid stimulating hormone and this peaks at midnight. The thyroid is stimulated to produce T4 (thyroxin), which spikes at 4:00 am. This is converted to the active thyroid hormone T3, which spikes at 5:00 am. T3 kicks the adrenals into life and the rising levels of adrenalin, cortisol and DHEA wake us up at 6:00-7:00 am. My guess is that it is the varying levels of all these hormones through the night that determine the proportion of non-REM to REM sleep, and this too is critical for good health.

Good thyroid and adrenal function are essential for good quality sleep. A further likely mechanism for sleep is the effect on core temperature. Indeed, there is a very clear relationship between the onset of sleep and falling core temperature and this is achieved by increasing blood flow to the skin, so heat is lost.

An hour of sleep before midnight is worth two after

Well known saying…and Mother was right again!

Early to bed and early to rise, makes a man healthy, wealthy, and wise.

Benjamin Franklin[‡] (17 January 1706 – 17 April 1790)

The quality of sleep

There are two recognisable types of sleep, called (1) rapid eye movement (REM) sleep and (2) non-REM sleep. We see a cycle of these every 90 minutes. Non-REM sleep comes first and during this time we sort through the experiences of the day and store the important ones, essential to survival, as memory. We then slip into REM sleep during which we dream, and problem solve. All sorts of odd connections are made. We start the night with a high proportion of non-REM to REM sleep and finish the night with more REM sleep. I suspect the proportions are determined by the changing levels of melatonin and thyroid and adrenal hormones which occur through the sleep cycle. It is easy to see how both sorts of sleep confer survival advantage. We do not want to clog up the brain with useless memories and we need to make lots of bizarre connections for problem solving.

[‡]**Historical note**: We do have Franklin to thank for bringing this well-known phrase into common usage. (My mother said this to me an awful lot during my teenage years, always with a strong emphasis on the 'wise': Craig) However, there are earlier versions, showing that indeed this wisdom has been known for hundreds of years. In *The Book of St Albans*, printed in 1486, we have: 'As the olde englysshe prouerbe sayth in this wyse. Who soo woll ryse erly shall be holy helthy & zely.' The Middle English word *zely* had numerous meanings in 1486 but foremost were 'auspicious' or 'fortunate'. So 'holy helthy & zely' meant 'wise, healthy and fortunate'. *The Book of St Albans* contains advice on hawking, hunting and heraldry with a chapter on fishing added in 1496.[2]

Just as the PK diet is non-negotiable, so too is sufficient sleep.

For non-REM sleep:

I consider that a man's brain originally is like a little empty attic, and you have to stock it with such furniture as you choose. A fool takes in all the lumber of every sort that he comes across, so that the knowledge which might be useful to him gets crowded out, or at best is jumbled up with a lot of other things, so that he has a difficulty in laying his hands upon it. Now the skilful workman is very careful indeed as to what he takes into his brain-attic. He will have nothing but the tools which may help him in doing his work, but of these he has a large assortment, and all in the most perfect order. It is a mistake to think that that little room has elastic walls and can distend to any extent. Depend upon it there comes a time when for every addition of knowledge, you forget something that you knew before. It is of the highest importance, therefore, not to have useless facts elbowing out the useful ones.

Sherlock Holmes from *A Study in Scarlet* by Sir Arthur Conan Doyle (22 May 1859 – 7 July 1930, buried 1930 and 1955[§])

For REM sleep:

The key to having good ideas is to get lots of ideas and throw out the bad ones.

Linus Pauling (28 February 1901 – 19 August 1994)

[§]**Literary note:** Conan Doyle was not a Christian, considering himself a Spiritualist, and so he was first buried on 11 July 1930 in Windlesham rose garden. His body was later reinterred together with his wife in Minstead churchyard in the New Forest, Hampshire.

And more from Thomas Dekker and, as Craig's wife, Penny, used to sing to their children every night:

Golden slumbers kiss your eyes,
Smiles awake you when you rise;
Sleep, pretty wantons, do not cry,
And I will sing a lullaby,
Rock them, rock them, lullaby.
Care is heavy, therefore sleep you,
You are care, and care must keep you;
Sleep, pretty wantons, do not cry,
And I will sing a lullaby,
Rock them, rock them, lullaby.

The Cradle Song by Thomas Dekker (c. 1572 – 25 August 1632),
English dramatist and pamphleteer

Homer, the (legendary) author of the epic poems, *The Odyssey* and *The Iliad*, knew that sleep was vital:

There is a time for many words, and there is also a time for sleep.

Homer,[¶] *The Odyssey*

[¶]**Historical note:** Homer was born sometime between the 12th and 8th centuries BC, possibly somewhere on the coast of Asia Minor. Very little is known about him, even whether he was really the author of these two poems. In fact, Homer may not even be a single person, but we digress. I agree with Homer about the importance of sleep. (Homer agrees with you, Sarah – Craig)

How to improve your sleep

Now see below for what you need to do to achieve the quantity, quality and timing of sleep for optimal health. I know I do not know all the answers to poor sleep (another steep learning curve) but you may find some below. Recently I have learned the importance of thyroid and adrenal hormones for good quality sleep. Am I not lucky? I am on such a journey[#] of interesting questions I know I shall never be bored.

The three steps to work through are:

1. Identify what is disturbing your sleep.
2. Get the physical essentials in place.
3. Get the brain off to sleep with a sleep dream.
4. Reinforce your sleep dream with a hypnotic if nothing else will do.

1. Identify what is disturbing your sleep

First think about what is disturbing your sleep. In order of likelihood think about: adrenalin, sleep apnoea syndrome, hormone issues, inflammation, detoxing and unpleasant symptoms such as pain.

Adrenalin

The commonest cause of disturbed sleep in Westerners is nocturnal hypoglycaemia because this spikes adrenalin levels.

Once PK-adapted, the brain happily runs on ketones and does not panic if sugar is not available.[♠] My dear friend (and co-author of our book *Green Mother*) Michelle eats PK.

[#]**Historical note:** *The Odyssey* is about a 'journey'. It is the second-oldest extant work of Western literature, *The Iliad* being the oldest, and as such it lays the foundation for much of Western thinking. A key point is that we are all on our own individual journeys of discovery.

[♠]**Footnote:** In 1992 Ranulph Fiennes and Dr Mike Stroud attempted an unassisted journey across Antarctica. They carried their own provisions with the most energy-dense food being high fat; they walked in permanent ketosis. Mike took regular blood tests and blood sugar levels fell below 1 mmol/l (reference range 4-6). They had no symptoms of low blood sugar because they were fuelling their mitochondria with ketones.

She breast-fed and weaned both her babies, Robyn and Etta, on a PK diet. Since 4 weeks of age both girls have never failed to sleep 11 hours, and by 2 months of age a solid 13 hours, at night. They continue to be great sleepers.

The issues with adrenalin are:

- Adrenalin derived from its mimics, such as caffeine and chocolate: Some people are very slow metabolisers, and these drugs can persist in the body for days.
- Adrenalin may come from stress.
- Alcohol is one of the most powerful disturbers of sleep. A large slug may get you off to sleep, but this triggers hypoglycaemia, adrenalin is then poured out and you wake in the middle of the night, wide awake, often unable to drop off again. Sigh! I love alcohol, but it is sleep loss that stops me drinking the lovely stuff. Indeed, all addictions disturb sleep.
- Adrenalin from the upper fermenting gut: The fermenting gut ferments carbs and, to a lesser extent, protein into many toxins, including alcohol, which have the potential to disturb sleep. The last meal of the day needs to be in the early evening, should be modest with no carbs and low protein but high in fibre and fat. Many find that fasting improves sleep quality.

Sleep apnoea syndrome

Stopping breathing is stressful and wakes you up. You may stop breathing because your airway is blocked, in which case your breathing is noisy, often with snoring (obstructive sleep apnoea). Alternatively, the brain forgets to trigger a breath, and this is called central sleep apnoea.

Causes of obstruction, and so snoring, include:

- obesity ('Pickwickian syndrome'♥)
- oedema (swelling) due to allergy or hypothyroidism
- undershot jaw with narrowing of the airways.

♥**Historical literary note:** Pickwickian syndrome is named after the character Joe (the 'fat boy') from Charles Dickens' novel *The Pickwick Papers*. Joe displayed all the characteristics of obstructive sleep apnoea. The first time that the term 'Pickwickian syndrome' was used is thought to be in a 1956 medical paper by Burwell et al.[3]

Causes of central sleep apnoea include poisoning by mycotoxins, chemicals and addictions.

Hormones

Hormones decline with age and parallel worsening sleep. It is melatonin that drives our sleep/wake cycle: 95% is produced in mitochondria in response to near infrared light for local antioxidant effects; 5% is made in the pituitary and this is released at night. Its production has a momentum of its own which explains why it takes a week to adjust to jet lag.

Melatonin does not make us sleepy, but we cannot sleep without it. With age our ability to make melatonin declines and, with that, our sleep quality declines in parallel. As described above, melatonin triggers the release of TSH which spikes at midnight, so thyroid hormones are produced, with T4 spiking at 4:00 am and T3 at 5:00 am. These kick the adrenals into life, with adrenal hormones and testosterone spiking at 6:00 am and this warms us up and wakes us up.

There are other vicious cycles here because poor sleep results in poor hormone production.

The dose of melatonin varies from 0.5 to 10 mg at night. Some worry they will get dependent on this, but I doubt it. There is no negative feedback pathway since production is dependent on light. So, to correct the hormonal environment:

- Get as much full-spectrum light as is possible by day. Sit outside or at least close to a window.
- Melatonin 0.5-10 mg at night.
- Then sort out your thyroid (see Chapter 7).
- And your adrenals (again see Chapter 7).

Inflammation

Inflammation occurs when the immune system is active for reasons of allergy, autoimmunity and/or infection. We all recognise the disturbed sleep of acute 'flu.

The immune system and the brain are remarkably similar. Both are sensitive, responsive, decision makers and are actively intelligent. Much inflammation starts with the fermenting gut, and where there is upper fermenting gut there is 'fermenting brain' – i.e. microbes in the gut may also be present in the brain where they ferment neurotransmitters into, amongst other things, amphetamine-like substances.[4] (See also Chapter 13 for the general approach to reducing inflammation.)

Detoxing

At night the supportive brain cells shrink by 60% to open up spaces for the glymphatics to clean up brain toxins, including the aforementioned amyloid proteins which drive dementia. I am not sure why this should disturb sleep, but it is very obvious clinically as part of detox reactions (see Appendix 2). Raising the head of the bed 6-12 inches (15-30 cm) facilitates this detox which occurs during deep sleep.

Unpleasant symptoms

Unpleasant symptoms include pain, shortness of breath, palpitations, reflux etc. In this event we need to work out the cause of the symptom. To cover all such is beyond the scope of this book; you need to see our book *Ecological Medicine.*

Get physical essentials sorted

Second, get the physical essentials in place. This includes: a comfortable bed, a dark, quiet room, temperature control, avoiding stimulants and getting timing right.

Knowing what may be causing the problem is essential to know what to do, but we must then actually do it!

> *Actions speak louder than words.*[**]

So these are the essentials to address:

1. A comfortable bed: We have been brainwashed into believing a hard bed is good

for us, so many people end up with sleepless nights on an uncomfortable mattress. Do whatever you need to distribute your weight evenly and avoid pressure points; memory-foam mattresses are often helpful as are water beds.

2. Raise the head of the bed 6-12 inches (15-30 cm): This is to facilitate the glymphatic drainage of the brain.
3. A dark room: The slightest chink of light landing on your skin will disturb your own production of melatonin. Have thick curtains or blackouts to keep the bedroom dark; this is particularly important for children. Do not switch the light on or clock-watch should you wake.
4. A quiet room: Do not allow a bed fellow who snores; you need different rooms.
5. Temperature control: Core body temperature falls at night, and this is an essential part of triggering sleep. Indeed, the mechanism that wakes us up is an increase in body temperature and that is driven by a spike of thyroid and adrenal hormones. Core body temperature is controlled by blood flow to the skin and heat is lost through sweating of this 'shell'. Wear cotton pyjamas that absorb sweat away from the skin to facilitate this. With no pyjamas, sweating leaves the skin icy-cold; this may be painful and that disturbs sleep. Meanwhile, falling body temperature is a powerful and essential trigger for sleep. This may explain why a warm bath helps – once out of the bath, heat is rapidly lost through the 'shell', so core temperature follows, and sleep is induced. Do not exercise hard before sleep; you will get too hot and stay hot.
6. The right balance of mental and physical activity: Expect to sleep better after a physically active day (within the bounds of pacing, see Chapter 9). Do not take problems to bed but remember that REM sleep problem solves – you may wake in the morning with the answer.[††]

[**]**Literary note:** This phrase possibly has its origins in the book of John in the Bible, where it is stressed that merely saying that you love someone is not the same as doing things for them. But in the form as above, it is attributed to Abraham Lincoln (President of the United States, 1861-1865, born 12 February 1809 – assassinated 15 April 1865) in 1856. Personally, I (Craig) prefer: 'A word spoken in season is like an Apple of Gold set in Pictures of Silver, and actions are more precious than words.' English Statesman, John Pym, 1584 – 8 December 1643.

[††]**Note:** Jacques Hadamard (8 December 1865 – 17 October 1963, French mathematician) wrote a book called *The Psychology of Invention in the Mathematical Field.* He included several examples of famous mathematicians dreaming about solutions, including Poincare. Poincare was called 'The Last Universalist' because it was said that he excelled in all fields of mathematics as it existed during his lifetime.

7. Avoid stimulants such as caffeine or adrenalin-inducing TV, arguments, phone calls, family matters or whatever before bedtime.
8. Get the timing right: As the day progresses, a 'pressure to sleep' builds up, so the longer we stay awake the greater is the need and desire to sleep. Over and above this sleep pressure throughout the 24 hours we also have a 90-minute sleep cycle. Learn to recognise this because you will have a much better chance of dropping off by riding the sleep wave. You may well feel such a sleep wave during the evening, perhaps feeling dozy whilst watching TV? It will come at the same time each evening. In winter, I eat supper at 6-ish, then crossword puzzle and telly. I take Nancy out ratting at 8:00 pm, am in bed by 8:15 pm at the latest, read, feel the sleep wave coming on at 9:00 pm, light out, sleep dream in place (see next)… and am gone. I have an alarm set for 6:00 am but it rarely goes off because I wake a few minutes prior. Remember, we hibernate in winter and need more sleep than in summer.
9. Have a regular rising time: Because of artificial lighting our internal clock runs late so there is a tendency to wake later every morning. It is well-recognised that a good (but counter-intuitive) way to improve sleep quality is to set the alarm clock for 30 minutes earlier and maintain that. I think this helps to mitigate the effects of artificial light.

3. Get the brain off to sleep with a sleep dream

Getting the physical things in place is the easy bit. The hard bit is getting your brain off to sleep. If you go to bed thinking about the previous day and planning the next day, then you have little chance of dropping off. However, the brain can be trained because, throughout life, it makes a million new connections every second. This means it has a fantastic ability to learn new things.

Getting off to sleep is all about developing a conditioned reflex. The best example of this is Pavlov's dogs. Pavlov was a Russian physiologist who showed that when dogs eat food, they salivate. He then 'conditioned' them by ringing a bell whilst they ate food. After two weeks of conditioning, he could make them salivate simply by ringing a bell. This of course is a completely useless conditioned response, but it shows us the brain can be trained, by association, to do anything.

Applying this to the insomniac, firstly one has to get into a mind set (sleep dream) which does not involve the immediate past or immediate future. That is to say, if you are thinking about reality then there is no chance of getting off to sleep.

> *You know you're in love when you can't fall asleep because reality is finally better than your dreams.*
>
> Dr Seuss, author of the *Cat in the Hat* books (1904 – 1991)

I do not pretend this is easy, but to allow one's mind to wander into reality when one is trying to sleep must be considered a complete self-indulgence. Treat your brain like a naughty child. It is simply not allowed to free wheel.

Find a sleep dream that suits you

If you think about real events then there is little chance of dropping off to sleep. You have to displace these thoughts with a sleep dream. It could be a childhood dream, or recalling details of a journey or walk, or whatever. It is actually a sort of self-hypnosis. What you are trying to do is to 'talk' to your subconscious. This can only be done with images, not with spoken language since your subconscious deals with emotions and feelings. I dream that I am a hibernating bear, snuggled down in my comfortable den with one daughter in one arm, the other in the other, and Nancy at my feet. Outside the wind is howling and the snow coming down and I am sinking deeper and deeper down...

Learning a sleep dream is a bit like riding a bicycle – it looks impossible at a distance but with a bit of practice becomes easy. Your brain will try to convince you that a sleep dream is not working, but that is just because the brain likes to free wheel, especially if you are naturally hypervigilant.

If you do wake in the night, do not switch the light on and do not get up and potter round the house or you will have no chance of dropping off to sleep. Use your sleep dream again.

4. Reinforce your sleep dream with a hypnotic if nothing else will do

If you cannot get the sleep dream to work, then reinforce this conditioning with a hypnotic. The idea here is that you take a sleep pill *and* do the sleep dream; you apply the two together for a period of 'conditioning'. This may be a few days or a few weeks. The brain then learns that, when it gets into that particular mindset, it will go off to sleep. Use of the medication should become unnecessary.

Medication for sleep

All sleep medications work only in the short term. They buy you a window of sleep for difficult times but are not a long-term solution. Use the window of time to really address underlying causes. As short-term remedies, consider:

- Nytol (diphenhydramine 50 mg): This is a sedating antihistamine available over the counter. The dose is 0.5-2 tablets at night. This is long acting so don't take it in the middle of the night or you will wake feeling hung-over.
- Valerian root 400 mg (1-4 capsules) at night. This is a herbal preparation which is shorter acting and can be taken in the middle of the night.
- Kava kava: This in not available in UK, Poland or the Netherlands but is in the USA and many other countries. In Australia supply is regulated.

It is vital to combine any of the above with a good sleep dream and all the interventions in this chapter. Do not use the medication without these interventions, otherwise tachyphylaxis (a decrease in response) will result.

Having said that, I have some patients who can only sleep with a prescription hypnotic. For some this results from decades of hypervigilance and PTSD, for others I suspect viral damage to the sleep centre of the brain. What characterises these few is their need for such medications remains constant and tachyphylaxis (progressive decrease in response) does not occur. In these particular cases, I am always asked about addiction. My experience is that this is rare, especially if drugs are used as above to develop a conditioned reflex or to treat pathologically awful sleep.

One has to distinguish between addiction and dependence. We are all dependent on food, but that does not mean we are addicted to it. We are all dependent on a good night's sleep for good health and may therefore become dependent on something to achieve that. This does not inevitably lead to addiction. Addiction is a condition of taking a drug excessively and being unable to cease doing so without other adverse effects. Stopping your hypnotic may result in a poor night's sleep but hopefully little more than that. This is not addiction but dependence. We know that taking prescription hypnotics for years is a risk factor for dementia. But then so is insomnia. I am not sure where the balance lies. But if it were me…? Well, I would take the sleeping pills and put in place everything else to protect against dementia. For me, sleep is an essential, not a luxury.

Table 8.1 summarises the causes of and possible treatments for sleep problems.

Table 8.1: Common causes of disturbed sleep and how to tackle them

Symptom	Mechanism	Treatment
Poor quality sleep	Lack of raw materials to make the necessary neurotransmitters	Tryptophan 8-12 g daily – it is very safe (see 'The Prozac story' below from our book *Ecological Medicine*)
'I just wake up as if it's morning, but it's 2:00 am'	Adrenalin from nocturnal hypoglycaemia (adrenalin is the usual stimulus for normal waking)	PK diet
	Ketogenic hypoglycaemia – i.e. fat burning using adrenalin instead of thyroid hormones	Sort out the underactive thyroid (see Chapter 7)
	Alcohol is a major cause of hypoglycaemia since it stimulates insulin release directly	Take care with alcohol Treat the fermenting gut or 'auto-brewery syndrome'
	The adrenalin of post-traumatic stress syndrome	Block this with a herbal beta blocker such as hawthorn 300 mg to 900 mg at night or propranolol 20 mg

Table 8.1 *Cont'd*

Symptom	Mechanism	Treatment
	Inadequate hormones or poor timing of their release	As above: melatonin Sort out your thyroid and adrenals (see Chapter 7)
	May be a detox reaction	See Appendix 2: DDD reactions
Sleep apnoea: obstructive	Obstruction may be due to: Obesity Allergy Hypothyroid (underactive) Undershot jaw Mouth breathing	PK diet – if this alone does not reduce weight then do the 5:2 diet; this never fails. Lower exposure to allergens. Correct thyroid hormone levels. See a good osteopath. See Chapter 6: Oxygen and do the breathing exercises, and tape your mouth shut for when you sleep
Sleep apnoea: central	Central sleep apnoea can result from neurological damage due to: mycotoxins (from moulds/fungi), pesticides, VOCs, toxic metals	See Chapter 14
Too hot: Hot flushes and sweating	Menopausal: One becomes very sensitive to any temperature fluctuation and a slight heat rise can trigger a flush	Do not take female sex hormones. Work on temperature control. All the above helps greatly to mitigate flushes, but cure not guaranteed
	The body trying to run a fever to deal with chronic low-grade infection	See Chapter 15 as the starting point to treat any chronic infection
Symptoms such as pain, wheeze, itching, restless legs	Allergy to food and/or gut microbes	See Chapter 13 for the general approach to reducing inflammation. Start the PK diet
Gut symptoms such as reflux, indigestion	Upper fermenting gut	PK diet. Vitamin C 5 g (or to bowel tolerance) plus Lugol's iodine 15% 3 drops at night

Symptom	Mechanism	Treatment
Constitutionally hard-wired for hypervigilance	Previous psychological trauma such as childhood bullying or abuse	Counselling Hypnotics may be helpful in the short term
Neurological damage...which may or may not also cause central sleep apnoea	Past head injury Poisoning by chemicals Pathology: ischaemia (stroke, dementia), prion disease, tumour	Do all the above Hypnotics may be helpful Try detox regimes (see Chapter 14)
Depression and many other brain conditions	I think depression is more often the result of poor sleep, not a cause	Improve energy delivery mechanisms Tryptophan 8-12 g daily – it is very safe (See 'The Prozac story' below from our book *Ecological Medicine*

The Prozac story

Tryptophan, an amino acid, is an effective antidepressant and was widely used on NHS prescription during the 1980s. It is the precursor for serotonin and probably fermented in the gut to such. We know the bacterium *E coli* does this. At last! A safe, effective, cheap, physiological treatment for low mood. You would think it impossible for Big Pharma to effectively abolish such a treatment? But tryptophan was a potential competitor to Big Pharma's new tranche of drugs, the SSRIs. A contaminated batch of tryptophan came onto the market from a single company in Japan, Showa Denko, and this batch alone produced a side effect – namely, eosinophilic myalgic syndrome. Big Pharma pounced on this opportunity and the propaganda that followed resulted in the effective banning of all the known-to-be-safe tryptophan preparations from the pharmacopoeia. Why? Follow the money.

And so to bed.

Expression often used at the end of his day's diary entries by Samuel Pepys, English MP and famous diarist (23 February 1633 – 26 May 1703)

Summary

- Good quantities (9 hours, perhaps a bit more in winter, less in summer) of good quality sleep are essential for recovery.
- If you are not getting good quantity and quality sleep, then work out why, and correct – namely:
  - Night-time adrenaline spikes causing hypoglycaemia – PK diet.
  - Sleep apnoea – look for mouth-breathing, allergy, hypothyroidism, undershot jaw, poisoning by mycotoxins, chemicals and addictions.
  - Hormone issues
    - Get as much full-spectrum light as is possible by day.
    - Melatonin 0.5-10 mg at night.
    - Then sort out your thyroid (see Chapter 7).
    - And your adrenals (see Chapter 7).
  - Inflammation: usually due to the upper fermenting gut – solution: PK diet.
  - Detoxing can cause sleeplessness – solution: raise the head of the bed by 6-12 inches (15-30 cm) to help the glymphatics and so facilitate detoxing.
  - Other unpleasant night-time symptoms – work out the cause (see our book *Ecological Medicine*.
- Get the basics in place:
  - comfortable bed
  - dark room
  - raise the head of the bed to aid detoxing during the night
  - have as quiet a room as possible
  - keep the temperature right for you to sleep – not too hot
  - do not take problems to bed
  - if you can exercise during the day, this will help
  - avoid stimulants like caffeine, TV, arguments etc before bedtime
  - have a regular bedtime and rising time.
- Develop your own sleep-dream and use it every night.
- If the combination of all this does not give you good quantity and quality sleep, then use the supplements and medications as indicated above.

Chapter 9

Pacing and the right sort of exercise

A good rest is half the work.

Yugoslavian proverb

How beautiful it is to do nothing and then rest afterwards.

Spanish proverb

Much old wisdom, such as in these old proverbs, about resting and pacing has been lost in the hubbub of modern life.

Pacing is all about spending energy wisely. We all lie on an energy spectrum, and I am to an elite athlete what a CFS/ME/LC sufferer is to me. We all have a certain bucket of energy (I will use this analogy many times) available to us and, for an elite athlete to overtrain is as dangerous as it is for a CFS/ME/LC sufferer not to pace. The characteristic symptom is delayed fatigue and, as detailed in Chapter 2, this is like borrowing energy from a loan shark – one ends up stuck in an energy trap.

In the early stages of recovery pacing is essential. We all know that exercise is good for our health, but that is only the case when energy delivery mechanisms are working. Many get into chronic fatigue because they have lived their life on adrenalin, burnt the candle at both ends and achieved at the expense of their health. For such people, much of the difficulty is letting go of the guilt of having to rest and pace. They need a personality change. Resting and pacing have to become seen as an 'intervention' in their own right, a part of the overall package required for recovery. They are not something 'to be fitted in' when you can – they are essential. You will *not* get better unless you learn to rest and pace well. And if you ever do feel guilt, then remember that, generally, the idle do not get fatigue syndromes.

Imagine that a normal healthy person has £1000 worth of energy to spend in a day. The CFS/ME/LC sufferer only has £100. What is more, this has to be spread out throughout the day in such a way that there is £20 'change' at the end. This allows energy for healing and repair, overnight. You initially have to do less in the short term in order to achieve more in the long term.

A fatigue-ometer would be a very useful gadget to make people pace; until such a device is available, we have to listen to our body.*

How to reduce energy expenditure

To recover we have to find ways to reduce energy expenditure. And yes, it is boring to have to do this, but also essential.

By 'rest', I mean complete mental, physical and emotional rest from exercise, visitors, telephone calls, reading, computers, talking, child-minding, noise and TV. All the above count as activities which have to be carefully rationed through the day. Also, if you feel yourself 'waiting' until your 'rest period' is done, so that you can get on with other things, then you are not really resting at all – you are marking time, so that, in your head, you can say to yourself that you *have* rested. You need to 'switch everything off'.

- Rest lying down: When you stop, use a recliner chair to lie horizontally because this reduces the work of the heart. (It is much harder work to push blood round a vertical body, up hill and down dale, than when horizontal, with everything on the flat.)

*__Footnote:__ In Craig's case, he literally does 'listen' to his body – his tinnitus! He suffers with this constantly and has done so since the early 1990s. The higher the pitch, the greater the urgency there is for him to take a rest.

- Do things in short bursts. You will be more efficient if you do things for 10-40 minutes (whatever your window of time is), then rest for the same length of time. I had one patient who could only walk 30 metres, but by walking 15 metres and resting, then going on again, she got up to walking a mile a day without delayed fatigue.
- Vary your activity: This applies to the brain as well as the body – for example, listening to the radio or music uses a different part of the brain to watching TV. Washing up (sitting on a high stool, please) uses different muscles to walking.
- Do things by the clock: We are creatures of habit, and the physical body likes things to happen on a regular basis; ask any farmer who keeps animals – they thrive on routine. Sleep and eat at regular times and pace activities so you do about the same every day and during the same time slots. I know that life has a habit of getting in the way of this ideal, but as a general principle, stick to it.
- Have a proper after-lunch rest: You should have a proper rest, perhaps when you actually go to bed, regularly in the day, even on days when you feel well. Ideally sleep. Homo sapiens evolved in hot climates where it is normal to have a siesta in the afternoon. Most people experience an energy dip after lunch. Young babies and older people return to this more normal sleep pattern, and ill people should do the same. An afternoon sleep is normal. I do it. It is called power-napping.
- Do not overdo things on a day that you feel well. Short-term symptoms can be misleading.
- Be careful with adrenalin: This temporarily masks the symptoms of over-doing it and can lead one astray. Adrenalin is false energy.
- Do not live life on the edge: A useful analogy is that CFS/ME/LC sufferers often live life on the edge of a cliff. A minor stress will tip them off the edge and down to the beach below; it is then a hard climb back. We should walk back from the edge onto the grassy slope. If we fall on this grassy slope, then we will not hurt ourselves and it is a small business to pick ourselves up and go again.

How to reduce energy expenditure: Prioritise, get organised and accept help

To reduce energy expenditure on routine activities:

- Apply for benefits (see Appendix 4 if you are based in the UK). Money helps a lot!
- List the 10 most important things in your life in descending order of preference. Then scrub out and cancel the bottom half.
- Do not be house-proud. Get a cleaner and dish washer if you can afford to. Give up ironing – it's a nonsensical, energy-sapping waste of time and energy. Ironing came into fashion to kills nits and fleas in the seams of clothes and had a purpose once. I don't iron.
- Accept offers of 'meals on wheels' from others.
- Shop online so food is delivered.

Summary: The 10 commandments for reducing energy expenditure

In a nutshell, the 10 commandments[†] for reducing energy expenditure are:

1. Thou shalt not be perfect nor try to be.
2. Thou shalt not try to be all things to all people.
3. Thou shalt leave things undone that ought to be done.
4. Thou shalt not spread thyself too thin.
5. Thou shalt learn to say 'No'.
6. Thou shalt schedule time for thyself, and for thy supporting network.
7. Thou shalt switch off and do nothing regularly.
8. Thou shalt be boring, untidy, inelegant and unattractive at times.
9. Thou shalt not even feel guilty.
10. Thou shalt not be thine own worst enemy, but thine own best friend.

[†]**Footnote:** Credit for this wonderful list goes to my patient, Sylvia Waites.

Pattern of recovery

People come to me feeling ill and having no energy. They push themselves to do things until the lactic acid pain is so awful that they are forced to stop. They are constantly fatigued and in pain.

The stages of recovery as listed below will not be a linear progression for everyone, maybe for no-one! There will be setbacks, and things will be very bumpy at times, and you may not 'fit' into a particular stage completely, but I do think it is very useful to have these stages listed out because then you can gauge roughly where you are and what you should, or should not, be doing.

The first stage: You start feeling awful. Then there are windows of improvement which arise as you learn to pace well. You start to see windows of time when you feel better (but cannot do more). These may just be a few hours initially, or a day or two. At this stage, do not be tempted to do more activity – that will just postpone your recovery and complicate things. The trouble is the very personality that often gets people into CFS/ME/LC does not help them to get out of it. Many CFS/ME/LC sufferers have a little devil on their shoulder that beats them up every time they try to rest.

The second stage: You feel fine doing nothing; you feel completely well whilst doing absolutely nothing. The reason why it is so important to get to this stage is because that is the best test of how the body is functioning. It is a measure of lactic acid in the body; if you get that lactic acid again, then you are slipping into anaerobic metabolism, which is back to loan-shark days (see page 8).

The third stage: You feel fine doing nothing every day. This stage is arrived at when you feel absolutely fine doing absolutely nothing (and of course this never really happens in real life because life has a habit of getting in the way) *and* this level of wellness is maintained for some days or, even better, weeks. That is to say, your level of wellbeing becomes established, more robust and less susceptible to the fluctuations of everyday life. Suddenly you start to have a future and your horizons expand. Then you can move into the fourth stage.

The fourth stage: Now you can do more. IT IS ABSOLUTELY ESSENTIAL

THAT the third stage has been reached before attempting this. Carefully start a very gradual process of doing more. The deal is that you are allowed to increase your activity, which may be mental or physical, on the grounds that you feel fine the next day. I do not mind people feeling tired at the end of the day. That is physiological and helps one to have a good night's sleep. However, if the fatigue is delayed and so you wake up the next morning feeling exhausted as a result of the previous day's exertions, then you have overdone things and you have to pull back. IT IS ESSENTIAL THAT YOU *LISTEN* and DO PULL BACK. OTHERWISE YOU RISK A RELAPSE AND RETURNING TO AN EARLIER STAGE OF THE PROCESS. This explains why there is no standard program of gradually doing more because however much you can or cannot do depends entirely on how you feel. So long as you continue to feel well and do not get delayed fatigue, then the process of doing more can be continued. But always go very gradually so as not to risk the gains that have been made. During all this time it is very important to hold the whole regime of diet, sleep, supplements, detoxing etc together. Improvement is not an excuse to relax the regimes.

The fifth stage: Additional exercises to restore numbers of mitochondria. Once you get to a stage where you feel well all the time and activity levels are acceptable, then you can start to do exercises to increase the numbers of mitochondria and so improve your cardiovascular fitness – see opposite for how to do this. AGAIN, DO NOT ATTEMPT THIS UNTIL STAGE FOUR HAS BEEN WELL ESTABLISHED, OTHERWISE A RELAPSE MAY BE A RISK. And again, IT IS ESSENTIAL THAT YOU *LISTEN* and DO PULL BACK if necessary.

The sixth stage: Balance up the regime with lifestyle. Now you can really start to have a life. You have the energy to spend on having fun. If you reckon that you have the energy of people of your age, then perhaps you can do a deal with the devil and take some liberties with the regimes. But for many, including me, the regimes are for life. As we age, we all get a chronic fatigue syndrome of sorts. It is pretty obvious why this is the case: energy levels are dictated by mitochondrial performance, and so too is the ageing process. The very interventions I recommend to treat chronic fatigue syndrome all slow the normal ageing process and prevent disease and degeneration. So, as we age, we can stay just as fit and just as well, but we must work much harder at it. Recovery is not a battle but a war. It is a war we all know we shall lose eventually, but if I lose my war aged 100[‡] then I will settle for that. The ageing process is also partly determined by micronutrient and antioxidant status. Like an old car, with age the friction in the system increases and that is paralleled by our need for micronutrients. Vitamin B12 is a common deficiency and there is no doubt that some people feel a lot better for the odd B12 jab. You might think that this is evolutionary nonsense since primitive man did not need B12 injections, but then on the other hand, by the age of 60,[§] most of us are on the evolutionary scrap heap and so evolutionary rules do not apply!

Long term: Knowing the above, I can say with confidence to my CFS/ME/LC sufferers that once they get on the regimes, not only should they improve, but their best years could be ahead of them and their risk of developing the diseases associated with the ageing process (cancer, dementia, heart disease etc) will be substantially reduced. I am greedy – I want the best quality of life for as long as possible – so I too observe all the regimes I impose on my CFS/ME/LC sufferers. This also helps me to understand how difficult these regimes are.

The right sort of exercise (the fifth stage, as above)

Humans, along with all other mammals, evolved living physically active lives. For herbivores this meant gentle aerobic activity pottering along and grazing. For carnivores, much of life would be spent sleeping or pottering around. But for both there would be occasions when maximum energy output was needed, either for a predator to run down a prey, or for a prey to escape from a predator. To survive such, both parties need to be physically fit. Perhaps once a week there will be a predator-prey interaction[¶] – the predator must run for her life to break her fast, the prey must run for his life to avoid

[‡]**Footnote:** As I write I am also caring for an old boy who fought in the Navy through the Second World War and wrote a fabulous book about his experiences, *A Home on the Rolling Main*. I feed him a PK diet and all the supplements. He is fit and well and his mind is as sharp as a tack – he is a great raconteur. This year, 2023, we have celebrated his 101st birthday.

[§]**Note from Craig:** I read this having recently celebrated my 60th birthday – on Christmas Day 2022.

becoming breakfast! In doing so, both parties will be pushed to their maximum physical output and will switch into anaerobic metabolism, with the production of lactic acid.

This is a key biochemical point because it is lactic acid that stimulates the growth of new mitochondria (thereby creating a bigger engine) and it is more mitochondria that give us bigger muscles. We know that poor health and the ageing process are both accompanied by loss of muscle. Getting into anaerobic metabolism is all we need to do to maintain muscle power *and* cardiovascular fitness. I learned this from Dr Doug McGuff and John Little in their book *Body by Science – a research-based programme for strength training, body building and complete fitness in 12 minutes a week.*[2]

Thanks to their work, we can now see how to exercise most efficiently. We do not want to do so much that we wear out our body. (This is what happens with so many athletes – most runners are carrying injuries, many are fit but not healthy.) The principle is to do slow powerful exercises for no more than 90 seconds until muscles go weak and ache with lactic acid burn. This is all that is required to get fit and stay fit. This approach makes perfect evolutionary sense. I do not see badgers and foxes trotting round my hill every morning to get fit.

Which exercises to do

My PBs (see page xvi) need exercises which require no equipment and little time. This is what I suggest:

1. Press ups. Start doing these with your knees on the ground. As you get stronger, one knee comes off the ground for each five press ups. As you get stronger, both knees can come off the ground. Do as many press ups as you can until you cannot do another one, your muscles are aching and your heart is going at 120 beats per minute

¶**Mathematical aside:** Predator-prey interactions are a fascinating topic in Mathematical Biology. It is all about relative rates of predation and reproduction; in a beautiful piece of mathematics, one can show what naturalists have known for centuries – that there is a point of equilibrium between predator and prey where numbers of each remain stable. Of course, add in multiple prey and multiple predators and unexpected events (e.g. prey- or predator-specific pathogens) and things become much more complicated and even more exciting![1]

(bpm). This will take 45-90 seconds. No longer. Then rest.

2. Squats. Stand sideways in and hang on to a door frame for balance. Bend your knees to go as low as you can – ideally onto your haunches. Stand up. Do as many as you can until you cannot do another one, your muscles are aching and your heart is going at 120 bpm. This will take 45-90 seconds. No longer. Then rest.

And that is it!

Do these first thing in the morning, every morning so they become part of your daily routine. This is all you need to do to have sufficient strength and fitness for normal human activities.

Many people kid themselves that they are getting fit by pottering along on the flat, but it is the old story – no pain, no gain. It is lovely fun and great for the brain to be out in Nature walking, gardening, swimming, cycling or whatever, but you need a brief window of time when the muscles ache, the heart rate gets to 120 bpm, and you are puffing and blowing to make any real gains.

Craig's experience regarding resting and pacing

When I first consulted with Sarah back in 2001, I had quite a few tests done, and then shortly afterwards I received a letter from her. This letter made me cry… tears of joy. It was the first time, after having been ill for eight years, that any doctor had told me about things in my body that were not working as they should have been. All previous doctors had given me a clean bill of health, even though I felt so terribly ill, and couldn't really function at all. In effect, this letter was the first validation of my illness, and, actually, it was also a validation of me.

The detail is not important but, for example, Sarah had isolated that my magnesium levels were very low, that my adrenals were not functioning properly, that I had high levels of harmful bacteria, yeast, and some parasites in my gut, and so on. Later we found out that chronic Epstein Barr virus (EBV – mononucleosis or glandular fever) infection and mercury poisoning were also big players. The road map was less complete in 2001 than it is now, but even then, Sarah knew 1000% more than any other doctor I had/have ever met before or since.

Nowadays, I think Sarah tests less than in those early days. She has learnt that the road map, as detailed in this book, will work for, and is needed by, most CFS/ME/LC sufferers, and that tests are expensive, and many sufferers are PBs, and that testing will only confirm what she already knows.

Now, much as I had tears of joy at Sarah's letter, I also had tears of frustration. Penny and I were PBs then. We are slightly less PBs now. And as I looked down the list of suggested interventions, I knew I could not afford all of them, maybe only just a few. For context, at this time, Penny was not working, and our two children, Gina and Conor, were young, and growing, and seemed to need new pairs of shoes every week. We were on benefits; actually we were a little better off than most in our circumstances because we received grants from both the Chartered Accountants' Benevolent Association and the Teachers' Benevolent Fund, but all the same, our financial position was precarious. As an example, our Building Society required an 'Income and Expenses' account every two weeks so that they could decide how much we should pay to them each month or else they would repossess our home. Penny was bringing up our two children and looking after bedridden me, so the job of producing an Income and Expenses account every two weeks quite rightly fell to me. So, I allocated 10 minutes of brain power to this task every morning, in bed obviously, as I was bedridden at this time. Doing this meant that in two weeks, I could produce what was required. My Income and Expense accounts were handwritten and always handed in on time – in one way, I was quite proud of them. However, I am sure that this situation did not do my fatigued adrenals much good.

But here is the point – included in Sarah's letter was a paragraph giving advice on resting and pacing. So, what was so important about that?

- Sarah mentioning the importance of resting and pacing validated what I had been forced to do by my illness, but more than that, it motivated me to be more focused on resting and pacing. I now saw it as part of my overall treatment package rather than something that the ME had imposed on me. In a single stroke of her pen, Sarah had changed resting and pacing from a 'negative' thing to a 'positive' thing.
- Money was tight but I could do resting and pacing! So, I could start SOMEWHERE.

- As I rested and paced better, and saw it as a positive thing, Penny needed to do less for me, because I began to feel a little better. This meant she could get a part time job and earn some money – good for her social and mental health. Also good for our bank account, and good for my adrenals too!
- In turn, this meant we could afford some of the other things that Sarah had suggested – so we put the diet into place.
- Again, I got a little better and, with the diet in place, Penny could increase her hours, we had more money and so could do the next thing as suggested by Sarah.

Rather clumsily perhaps, what I am trying to say is that resting and pacing are 'free' and so can be done by all. I do understand that for some sufferers, not only is money tight but also, so is time (if they are working), and so in that sense, there may be a 'cost' associated with resting (lost income for those hours resting), but there is no 'direct' cost, as such. Done well, it can kickstart your recovery and you can spiral (slowly) upwards just as I have described above. Of course, I was so lucky to have Penny, and lucky in so many other ways, and I don't mean to trivialise the situation that other sufferers find themselves in, but I hope you get the point – no matter how bad things are, I truly believe that there is always hope for recovery, and it often starts with proper rest and pacing.

One block I had to proper rest and pacing was a sense of guilt. I felt I should be doing more to help Penny, or that I should (somehow) be earning money and not be 'idle'. Whenever I felt in danger of breaking Commandment Number 9 above: Thou shalt not even feel guilty, I remembered a word that my Latin teacher had taught me – otiation[#] ('the state of being at leisure or doing nothing') – and somehow the fact that I was 'otiating' made me feel better about it. I think that, for many sufferers, guilt is a big block to proper rest and pacing, and so if you do feel in danger of breaking Commandment Number 9, please find your own way of countering that; it is perhaps the most crucial of Sarah's 10 Commandments. Ultimately, resting and pacing will help your recovery, and this will help all things. So, I also used to say to myself: 'Resting and pacing are not just

[#]**Linguistic note:** Otiation derives from the Latin word *otium* ('ease, leisure, freedom from business'), a word of unknown etymology, and I always thought it was quite fitting that the origin was unknown – less work for the poor students, learning its declension, origins etc.

for me. They make Penny's life easier too because I will feel better, and so she will then have to do less for me,' and so on.

In essence, by looking after yourself, you also look after the ones you love.

Summary

- Resting and pacing are essential to recovery and require the sufferer to learn how to listen to their body.
- Learn to look at resting and pacing as positive interventions rather than something that your illness has imposed on you.
- Doing things in short bursts, varying activity and having a regular routine all help.
- Build periods of rest, and even sleep, into that routine.
- Be careful with adrenaline – it can mask the fact that you are actually overdoing things. Adrenaline is false energy (see Chapter 7).
- Prioritise things, get help where you can, apply for benefits, and re-read the 10 commandments as above. Do NOT feel guilty about resting and pacing.
- Become familiar with the stages of recovery and plan what you do based on where you think you are within those stages.
- When ready, commence the exercises as described, but do be prepared to pull back if necessary. Do NOT push through.

Chapter 10

Myalgic encephalitis (ME) and long covid (LC): The symptoms of inflammation

Again I cannot over-emphasise the importance of the diagnoses 'ME' and 'LC' being clinical pictures and not true diagnoses – that is, identification of what is really wrong. So many doctors and researchers are stuck in the paradigm of one symptom from one diagnosis leading to one treatment. They are still looking for 'the Cure', have been for decades and doubtless will continue to do so. We have to break things down into diagnostic chunks.

> **CFS** is the clinical picture that arises from poor energy delivery mechanisms.
>
> **ME** is the clinical picture that arises from poor energy delivery mechanisms AND inflammation (the immune system is busy).
>
> **LC** is ME which follows acute Covid infection and/or Covid-19 mRNA gene therapy 'vaccines'.

That LC is a 'subset' of ME that happens to follow acute Covid-19 and/or Covid-19 mRNA gene therapy, rather than, say, EBV infection, is *obvious* to me because I am a clinician and I have seen so many ME patients over the years – in excess of 8000. The science will take years to catch up and, dear reader, you don't have years to wait. However, if you would like some reassurance that we are indeed talking about the same clinical picture, please see the paper by Timothy Wong and Danielle Weitzer: 'Long COVID and Myalgic Encephalomyelitis/Chronic Fatigue Syndrome (ME/CFS) – A Systemic Review and Comparison of Clinical Presentation and Symptomatology', which concluded that: 'Twenty-one studies were included in the qualitative analysis. Long

COVID symptoms reported by the included studies were compared to a list of ME/CFS symptoms compiled from multiple case definitions. Twenty-five out of 29 known ME/CFS symptoms were reported by at least one selected long COVID study.'

The starting point for treatment is to improve energy delivery mechanisms – that is, all that has gone before, in Chapters 1-9. Now we have to ask why the immune system is overactive and what we can do about that.

The symptoms of inflammation

The symptoms of inflammation occur when the immune system is busy. They may be local or general:

- Local symptoms include pain, redness, swelling, heat and loss of function. These include clinical pictures such as irritable bowel syndrome, migraine, arthritis, fibromyalgia, asthma, myocarditis, arteritis, polymyalgia, urticaria, eczema, rhinitis, nephritis, cystitis, prostatitis and much more.
- General body symptoms include malaise (feeling 'flu like), possibly fever, widespread pain and, again, loss of function.
- Inflammation in the brain results in sickness behaviour: lethargy, depression, anxiety, malaise, loss of appetite, sleepiness, hyperalgesia, reduction in grooming, and failure to concentrate. Sickness behaviour is a motivational state that reorganises our priorities to allow us to cope with infectious pathogens, allergies or autoimmunity. Again and just for clarity, it is not a psychological illness.

The problem with inflammation is that the symptoms are non-specific and may give us few clues about the cause. This means we have to start with the clinical picture and go through the likely causes. For much more detail see the bible, whoops, I mean our book *Ecological Medicine.*

The overall strategy to put out these inflammatory fires is to:

- identify the cause and remove it (turn off the gas to the cooker). This is about good detective work and perhaps some tests.
- extinguish the inflammatory fire (smother the flames) – with the general approach to

reducing inflammation (see Chapter 13).

- but if that is not enough, reprogramme the immune system (Chapter 19) and learn not to make the same mistake again. This is not easy – old habits die hard!

Summary

- ME is CFS plus inflammation (i.e. the immune system is busy).
- LC is ME following acute covid infection and/or covid 19 mRNA gene therapy 'vaccines'.
- In addition to all the treatments suggested in Chapters 1-9, we now need to add in more treatments to deal with this inflammation by:
    - identifying the cause of the inflammation and removing it.
    - extinguishing the inflammation.
- And if that is not enough, we may have to reprogram the immune system.
- Read on!

Chapter 11

Overview of the mechanisms of inflammation and how to fix them

There are many possible causes of inflammation* ranging from infections, both acute and chronic, to allergic reactions to food, pollen, pollutants, electromagnetic fields, chemicals, and also allergy to microbes arising from the fermenting gut. Fixing these inflammatory responses can be difficult and often requires a multi-pronged approach, including the implementation of the Groundhog regimes (Appendix 1), maybe adopting a carnivore diet (page 25), and possibly reprogramming the immune system with micro-immunotherapy (Chapter 19). Read on and digest the detail. This is a crucial area for your recovery.

***Linguistic note:** The word 'inflammation' derives from the Latin verb *inflammare*, which combines *flammare* ('to catch fire') with the Latin prefix *in*, which means 'to cause to'. This is a good description of inflammation in the body. There is an interesting quirk in the English language here – the words 'inflammable' and 'flammable' mean the same thing in modern usage – that is, 'capable of catching fire'. This is contrary to 'standard' English where the addition of 'in' as a prefix normally means 'not' as in, for example, 'inactive'. So, how did this arise? The story goes that in 1813, a scholar translated the Latin *flammere* to 'flammable' and after that 'flammable' came into common usage. The usage of 'inflammable' is decreasing, partly because many government regulations require 'flammable' to be used on products and official literature to avoid confusion, and 'non-flammable' is now the designated negative. Anyway, less of government regulations and back to the body….

Table 11.1: The clinical pictures of various types of inflammation and the actions needed to fix them

Clinical picture	Likely cause	Action
Acute infection – prevention is better than cure![†]	Virus, bacteria, fungi	Groundhog Acute (see Appendix 1). Especially vitamin C, 10 g hourly to bowel tolerance (see Chapter 4, page 44 for the details of bowel tolerance). In the event of respiratory symptoms sniff iodine. Rest, keep warm, do not suppress symptoms
Headache or migraine Gut pain, diarrhoea/ constipation Mood swings Muscle cramp Eczema, asthma, rhinitis	Allergy to food	Do not bother with food allergy tests – they are expensive, with too many false positives and negatives. PK diet. If the symptom does not settle then do a carnivore diet for up to one month, possibly less, until the symptom settles (see Chapter 4). Then bring in new foods one at a time, one day at a time. The general approach to reducing inflammation (Chapter 13). Reprogram the immune system (Chapter 19)
	Pollen, dust, dander, mycotoxins	Avoid
	Pollutants e.g. volatile organic compounds (VOCs)	Avoid. Heating regimes (see Chapter 14)

[†]**Historical footnote:** Benjamin Franklin expanded on this idea when he said that: 'An ounce of prevention is worth a pound of cure.' Franklin (17 January 1706 – 17 April 1790), polymath and one of the Founding Fathers of the United States, was talking about fire prevention to fire-threatened Philadelphians in 1736, but his comments ring as true for disease prevention.

Table 11.1 *Cont'd*

Clinical picture	Likely cause	Action
	Pollutants e.g. toxic metals	Avoid. Get rid of these (see Chapter 14)
	Electromagnetic radiation	Avoid
Arthritis (rheumatoid, polymyalgia rheumatica, psoriatic, Reiter's, ankylosing spondylitis etc) Inflammatory bowel disease (IBD) Interstitial cystitis Chronic urticaria Asthma Glomerular nephritis Vasculitis Psychological and psychiatric disease	Allergy to microbes from the upper fermenting gut (also known as 'molecular mimicry')	Starve 'em out with a PK, possibly carnivore diet. Kill 'em with vitamin C, 5 grams in the morning and Lugol's iodine 15% 3 drops at night. The general approach to reducing inflammation (Chapter 13). Reprogram the immune system (Chapter 19)
Autoimmune disease – most often switched on by vaccination, but it runs in families	Autoantibodies	Autoantibody screening is helpful for diagnosis. Autoimmunity is easy to switch on but difficult to switch off – ditto above
Chronic malaise dating from an acute infection e.g. long Covid	Inadequate immune response to an acute infection so that it becomes chronic	The general approach to treating any chronic infection (see Chapter 15). DMSO, methylene blue, photodynamic therapy (Chapters 16, 17, 18)
	If the general approach to treating any chronic infection does not do the trick, then try:	Tests to try to identify the infection and use specific antimicrobials. Viral screen at Armin laboratories. Bacterial screen at Armin laboratories (see Useful resources, page 303). Mycotoxin testing for fungal load (again, see Useful resources)
		The general approach to reducing inflammation (see Chapter 13)

There is much overlap between interventions to improve energy delivery mechanisms and inflammation. Addressing the former effectively helps to clear the murky clinical picture and makes it much easier to discern the cause of inflammation. And that of course has obvious implications for management.

Summary

- Inflammation arises from:
  - Acute infections
  - Allergy to food
  - Allergy to microbes
  - Allergy to pollen, dander, dust and pollutants (VOCs and toxic metals)
  - Mycotoxins
  - Electromagnetic radiation
  - Autoantibodies
  - Inadequate immune response leading to chronic inflammation.
- For the detail of treatments, see Chapters 13, 16, 17, 18 and 19. These include:
  - The general approach to reducing inflammation (Chapter 13)
  - DMSO, methylene blue, photodynamic therapy, micro-immunotherapy.

Chapter 12

Allergy and autoimmunity

Allergy and autoimmunity are immunological errors. The immune system is our standing army and essential to fight foreign invaders (viruses, bacteria, pathogenic fungi). Allergy is when we fight tourists (such as foods, animal dander and pollen) and we all know that is a rotten idea. Autoimmunity is civil war* – we turn on the self-destruct button to destroy our own tissues (as in Hashimoto's thyroiditis, pernicious anaemia, Addison's disease etc). That too is a rotten idea.

The immune system is easy to switch on but difficult to switch off. It is essential for our immune system armies to constantly be in the starting blocks and ready to swing into action at the first hint of infectious attack. This is lifesaving. We know that many cases of ME are triggered by an acute infection (typically Epstein Barr virus (EBV), acute Covid-19, Lyme disease, influenza and more) but that acute inflammation then fails to 'switch off'. This observation gives us the basic principles of preventing and treating chronic immune activation.

***Historical note from Craig:** One of the beauties of being married to an historian is that one picks up facts all through one's life that one would probably never come across otherwise. At her school, Penny is known as The Historical Google – she is 'old school' – she actually knows things. The English Civil War was brutal and, Wikipedia agrees with Penny here, that between 1638 and 1651, around 20% of all adult males in England and Wales served in the military. Approximately 4% of the total population died (this includes the two Bishops' wars, in Scotland) from war-related causes in the English Civil War, compared to around 2% in WWI. I have skirted round the Bishops' wars – my mathematical mind likes to keep things simple. So, yes, Civil War is a rotten idea. And that immediately triggers 'rotten boroughs', also learnt from Penny. But my digression has digressed and so I shall stop there.

Do not switch on the immune system without good reason

We prevent the immune system switching on without good reason in two ways: treat acute infection with 'Groundhog Acute' (see Appendix 1), and avoid the toxins that our immune system reacts to.

1. Treat acute infection with Groundhog Acute (see Appendix 1)

The principle of Groundhog Acute is to reduce the infectious load as quickly as is possible. Vitamin C to bowel tolerance (see Chapter 4: 10 grams (g) every hour to diarrhoea) massively reduces the infectious load in the gut (and 90% of infections access the body via the gut) and contact kills any microbes which remain. Sniffing iodine does the same in the respiratory tract. This reduces the work of the immune system to deal with any systemic invasion as the infectious load is substantially reduced. One still acquires natural immunity which is of course wholly desirable. A short, sharp, effective immune activation settles down quickly. The immune systems of our children should be so trained by being exposed to measles, mumps, rubella, chicken pox etc. With Groundhog Acute in place, not only is natural immunity achieved for life, but we know such acute febrile illnesses in childhood are protective against cancer and heart disease. Vaccines do not afford natural immunity for life nor protection against cancer and heart disease (see our book *Green Mother*).

A prolonged immune response to a high infectious load takes much longer to settle down. Post infectious syndromes lasting weeks are common; when they last months we call them myalgic encephalitis.

Always treat any acute infection with Groundhog Acute as prevention is better than cure.

2. Avoid toxic chemicals: heavy metals, pesticides, pollutants, addictions, prescription drugs, silicones

The immune system is switched on when it perceives a foreigner that has the potential to do harm. Heavy metals, pesticides, pollutants, addictions, prescription drugs, silicones are all harmful. The mechanism is as follows.

There is an inertia in the immune system, so it takes time to switch on. In the case of an acute infection, say measles, this inertia allows the measles virus to get ahead of the game and so measles illness results. Then this virus is killed and cleared away by inflammation. The immune system learns, so at a subsequent exposure to measles virus, the inertia has gone, and the virus is immediately killed. We call this immunity, and it is highly desirable.

Precisely the same principles apply to other such foreigners. In small amounts, the immune system perceives no danger and ignores the invader. In larger amounts, inflammation is switched on to kill and clear the foreigner. But many are tough molecules that cannot be broken down and cleared away, so the immune system goes on fighting

†**Personal note from Craig:** Reading Sarah's words above, I can categorically state that I am a textbook example. I fell ill with ME 'proper' on 15 March 1993 (the Ides of March) after a bout of influenza 'B'. I collapsed in London – and the rest of that story is told in my dedication to our book *Paleo-Ketogenic – The Why and the How*, if you're interested. I had, however, been suffering from a very mild chronic fatigue since 1982 after contracting EBV at university. I managed to lead a normal life between 1982 and 1993, gaining my degree, qualifying as a Chartered Accountant, marrying, working full time, and having two children. But I so wish I had known about Groundhog Acute back in 1982. In all likelihood, I would never have become ill with ME had I applied said Groundhog, and so I guess I would not be writing these words now. The advice I received from doctors at the time was woeful: after the EBV, the advice was to carry on exactly as before – late nights, parties, etc – with no attention to diet or anything really. I was given large doses of steroids 'to reduce the inflammation and get me back on my feet'. The advice after the 'flu B infection was to 'get back to work as soon as you can, or else you will get used to the "Life of Riley"'.

Riders to Personal note:

- The Romans marked the Ides of March with several religious observances but, probably more importantly, it was a deadline for the settling of debts. In 44 BC, it became notorious as the date of the assassination of Julius Caesar.
- 'Life of Riley' – this expression comes from a popular song of the 1880s, *Is that Mr Reilly?*, in which the title character describes what he would do if he suddenly became wealthy.

and chronic inflammation ensues. This inflammatory fire may start locally but then spreads systemically. We call this allergy, and it is highly undesirable. This inflammatory fire may result in autoimmunity when allergy to self is ignited.

Vaccines are especially good at switching on allergy and autoimmunity. They are a mixture of microbes, metals and other such toxins which activate the immune system with the potential to activate it inappropriately – against foods or self or perhaps friendly gut microbes. Vaccines are a double-edged sword. What really gave me the confidence to eschew them was the knowledge of the effectiveness of Groundhog regimes, especially Groundhog Acute to protect us from acute infection. These render vaccines largely irrelevant except for a few. (See our book *Ecological Medicine* for much more detail.) What I do know it that vaccines are a powerful trigger for myalgic-encephalitis (including long Covid).

How to switch the immune system off

Once the immune system has been switched on, switch it off by:

1. The general approach to reducing inflammation (see Chapter 13).
2. Specific approaches to reprogram the immune system (see Chapter 19).

Summary

- Allergy is where the immune system fights external allergens such as foods, animal dander and pollen. This is an error by the immune system – foods, animal dander and pollen do not represent a danger.
- Autoimmunity is where the immune system fights our own tissues. Again, this is an error by the immune system. Vaccines are the main cause.
- The immune system is easy to switch on but much harder to switch off.
- So, again, prevention is better than cure and it is best to avoid switching the immune system on in the first place:
  - Treat acute infection with Groundhog Acute.
  - Avoid vaccines.

  - Avoid toxic chemicals: heavy metals, pesticides, pollutants, addictions, prescription drugs, silicones.
- If the immune system has been switched on, then:
  - Apply the general approach to reducing inflammation (see Chapter 13).
  - Consider specific approaches to reprogramme the immune system (see Chapter 19).

Chapter 13

The general approach to reducing inflammation

The principles of treating inflammation are:

- Identify the cause and remove it (turn off the gas to the cooker).
- Extinguish the inflammatory fire* (smother the flames).

The UK National Fire Chiefs Association agrees when they write: 'All fires can be extinguished by cooling, smothering, starving or by interrupting the combustion process to extinguish the fire.'[1] In practice, these two principles of treatment are addressed together by the interventions listed below.

***Classical note from Craig:** I am reminded of a famous Latin palindrome involving 'fire': *'in girum imus nocte et consumimur igni*, 'We enter the circle at night and are consumed by fire.' This palindrome was intended to describe the behaviour of moths, who fly close to that which attracts them (flames) and are then consumed by them. Perhaps there is a parallel for us – we should avoid those things that 'attract' us and yet which lead to inflammation in our bodily systems: sugar, and other pro-inflammatory foods. But, in addition, we also have to be proactive and take positive action – e.g. with supplements, herbs etc as described below. This palindrome is also the title of a film by French Marxist filmmaker, Guy Debord. Perhaps there is a dark irony in the manner of his death, involving inflammation as it did. Debord died by suicide, by shooting himself through the heart. This suicide was, some say, brought on by a desire to end the suffering he endured from polyneuritis, a general inflammation of the peripheral nervous system. However, one cannot be sure; Debord had suffered from depression and alcoholism extensively throughout his life. Let us not be attracted by the flames and let us not be consumed by the fire! Read on.

Diet and gut function

- Do a paleo-ketogenic (PK) diet. Well, of course you are. When sugar is used as a fuel, many free radicals are produced, and this is pro-inflammatory. Not so with ketone fuels. The major food allergens are dairy products, gluten grains and yeast. The PK diet is a great start. Some need to do a carnivore diet, then identify food allergies by reintroducing foods one at a time, one day at a time (see Chapter 4).
- Tackle the upper fermenting gut. Microbes do pass from the gut into the bloodstream.[2] If these are friendly microbes from the lower gut that the immune system has been looking at for thousands of years, then they can be ignored and are excreted in urine (which is not sterile; the definition of a urine infection is having more than 10,000 microbes per ml). However, if we have unfriendly microbes from the upper gut, then they will get stuck at distal (faraway) sites and drive pathology. Examples include blood vessels (vasculitis and temporal arteritis), muscles (fibromyalgia and polymyalgia), joints (rheumatoid arthritis, ankylosing spondylitis, psoriatic arthritis) and brain (psychosis) (see our book *Ecological Medicine* for more detail). The starting point to tackle the upper fermenting gut is the PK diet; vitamin C, 5 grams (g) in the morning; and Lugol's iodine 15%, 3 drops at night (see Chapter 4).
- Consider probiotics. *Lactobacillus rhamnosus* and *plantarum* are of proven benefit. The best results are from live ferments (grow your own, which is the cheapest and the best option). To survive stomach acid, these microbes need some sugar – I suggest 0.5 tsp of the white stuff with a portion. This will feed them and power their proton pumps, which kick the acid out.[3]
- Sauerkraut. You can make your own; there is a recipe in our book *Paleo-Ketogenic – The Why and the How* or you can buy this from many suppliers (see Useful resources, page 303).
- Faecal bacteriotherapy. 90% of the immune system is associated with the gut and these mature, grown-up cells at the 'coal face' know what they must and must not react to. Immature 'adolescent' immune cells are released on a daily basis from the bone marrow into the bloodstream and they learn from the 'grown-ups' (i.e. the already existing immune cells). They learn to tolerate the status quo and become mature cells in their turn, and so immune memory is passed down through the generations and maintained in this way. This explains the mechanism of ongoing

immune tolerance to gut microbes and food – we ignore these friendly antigens and do not react against them as if they were foreigners. We learn to distinguish friend from foe. Thomas Borody improved 70% of his patients with ME, with 58% having a sustained response using faecal bacteriotherapy.[4, 4a]

Improve antioxidant status with micronutrients

Inflammation generates free radicals (for the boffins these are molecules with an unpaired electron) which have the potential to stick on to any other molecule and create biochemical havoc (for example, to stick to DNA and trigger a mutation). An antioxidant is any molecule that will neutralise such an unpaired electron and so quench a free radical. However, in the process of achieving such, the effectiveness of that molecule is lost. It has to be refreshed to become effective again. The body achieves this with a chain of molecules. This is akin to putting out a fire with a chain of people passing on buckets of water – we have a brave fire-fighter in the front row with second and third liners behind keeping her supplied. These include vitamin C to bowel tolerance and vitamin D 10,000 iu daily. You need to get above 160 nmol/l vitamin D for best anti-inflammatory effects. This may be achieved with 10,000 to 20,000 iu daily. Some physicians use much higher doses but in this event the level of serum calcium needs monitoring.

So, who are these wonderful characters who deal with these hot free radicals and electrons and flick them back to other catchers before they are finally quenched?

- The front-line grabbers include:
  - Inside mitochondria – co-enzyme Q 10, and manganese-dependent superoxide dismutase (SODase)
  - Inside cells – zinc, and copper-dependent SODase
  - Outside or between cells – extracellular zinc, copper, SODase, and glutathione peroxidase (which needs glutathione and selenium).
- The intermediate catchers include lots of molecules including many B vitamins, especially B12, vitamins A, D, E, K, and melatonin. All plants have their own system of antioxidants which we plant-eaters make use of. This means that all fresh, organic, raw foods will have an abundance of natural antioxidants.
- The final quencher of hot free electrons is vitamin C.

- Then we have iodine. This is a scavenger of free hydroxyl radicals, so further assisting all the above.

This system of catchers and quenchers (cripes – sounds like a game of quidditch![†]) has a numbers dimension. We need front-liners in microgram amounts, catchers in milligrams and the quencher vitamin C in gram amounts. All have to be present and correct in adequate amounts for this system to work effectively. The commonest deficiency is vitamin C. That is why the greatest need for any inflammation is vitamin C to bowel tolerance. So which supplements do we need to improve antioxidant status. Table 13.1 gives the details.

Table 13.1: The supplements we need to improve antioxidant status

Which supplement	Containing	To improve
Groundhog Basic multivitamins and minerals	Zinc 30 mg and copper 1 mg	Intracellular SODase Extracellular SODase
	Manganese 1 mg	Mitochondrial SODase
	Selenium 200 mcg (up to 500 mcg)	Glutathione peroxidase
	Methylcobalamin 5 mg (5000 mcg)	Vitamin B12[5]
	Vitamins A 2000 iu and E 50 mg	Vitamin A and E levels

[†]**Note from Craig:** Sarah is an avid reader of the Harry Potter series of books. I have never read them, although during my bedridden years, I did hear Penny read the first few books to my children, as bedtime stories, through the bedroom wall. It is so strange (and wonderful) what people like to read and what others don't. Harry Potter has never appealed to me, although I have now seen all the films, and secretly I quite like them. When I first read the words above, 'This system of catchers', my synaesthesia (experiencing one sense through another) kicked in and immediately I thought of *The Catcher in the Rye* (1951) by J.D Salinger (American author, 1919 – 2010). For me, this is a rare book because the mix of the shape of the words, the sounds of the words, the meanings of the words and the letters themselves lead to both the title and the author of this book having almost exactly the same 'mix' of synaesthetic colours. Having the title and author of a book 'match up' synaesthetically is very rare. In addition, this book has the magnificent line 'She was terrific to hold hands with.' I know – I'm a soppy git!

Which supplement	Containing	To improve
	Vitamin D 10,000 iu. (If you are off dairy and on no calcium supplements it is safe to take 20,000 iu daily. Also, it is safe to use 30,000 iu for three months, then reduce to 10,000 iu.) AND/OR Sunshine 1 hour daily	Vitamin D levels
	Vitamin C 5 g daily or to bowel tolerance	Vitamin C levels
Glutathione	Glutathione 250 mg (up to 500 mg)	Glutathione peroxidase Multitasks to help detox
Co-enzyme Q10	Ubiquinol 100 mg (up to 300 mg)	Co-Q10 levels
Iodine	Lugol's iodine 15% 3 drops	Iodine levels
Vegetables and berries in the PK diet	Natural antioxidants	All antioxidants

Quench the inflammatory fire

With herbs

The most important to take as a daily dose are:

- curcurmin (up to 2000 mg)
- ginger (up to 4000 mg)
- ashwaganda (up to 5000 mg)
- astragalus (up to 30 g)
- boswellia (up to 5 g)
- berberine (up to 3000 mg).

You may know instinctively what to take. If it smells and tastes good (addiction aside – we're not talking about sugar here) it will do good. Animals use scent to identify healing herbs – this is called zoopharmacognosy and, yes, I loved the book *Help Your Dog Heal Itself* by Caroline Ingraham.[6]

With essential oils

Again, if you like the smell, then it is probably good for you.

With minerals

- Magnesium 300 mg daily together with vit D 10,000 iu for its absorption.
- Alkalise the body with magnesium carbonate 5 g daily dissolved in water. Take this at least 90 minutes away from food as we need an acid stomach to digest food. This also supplies a dose of magnesium.
- Boron at least 3 mg and up to 20 mg daily. It has an multiplicity of anti-inflammatory actions.[7]

With low-dose naltrexone (LDN)

This is a popular and very safe way to treat any condition associated with inflammation. It is of proven effectiveness with a multiplicity of uses.[8] The idea here is to give a miniscule dose of the opiate-blocker naltrexone (start with 1 mg at night and build up to 4 mg), which has the effect of blocking the body's own production of endogenous opiates or endorphins. The body responds to this by ramping up its own production. Opiates are natural anti-inflammatories. For details of how to access LDN see my webpage listed in Useful resources (page 303).

Detox

Finally, we need to detox. We live in a toxic world, and we are all poisoned. We know all these poisons switch on inflammation and we must do all possible to reduce the load (see Chapter 14).

Summary

- Inflammation can be treated by:
  - identifying the cause and removing it.
  - extinguishing the inflammatory fire.
- Both of these are achieved by:
  - Eating a PK diet and getting rid of the fermenting gut.
  - Taking probiotics.
  - Eating fermented foods.
  - Maybe consider faecal bacteriotherapy (see page 129).
- Key also is getting antioxidant status up to scratch with:
  - the supplements listed above.
  - the herbs and essential oils listed above.
  - the minerals listed above.
  - consider using low-dose naltrexone (LDN) also.
- Detoxing (see Chapter 14).

Chapter 14

Detoxing

Get rid of toxic metals, pesticides, VOCs, prescription drugs, mycotoxins and more

Reduce your exposure to toxins

First, do your best to reduce your exposure to toxins. The main sources of these, in order of importance, are as listed in Table 14.1. I have included some references for these, but I am mindful that this book is written on a 'need to know' basis and is not a textbook of medical studies. At the same time, I am aware that references can sometimes help to give more impetus for action. In addition, on occasion I have referenced links to webpages on my website, where you will find further detailed references on that topic. If you are reading this as an ebook you will be able to go straight to the relevant page.

Table 14.1: The toxins to avoid

What	Why and How
Addictions: Sugar and fructose, smoking, vaping, alcohol, caffeine, cannabis etc	
Products of the upper fermenting gut (UFG)	Foods are fermented to toxins such as ethyl, propyl and butyl alcohols, D lactate, ammonia compounds, hydrogen, hydrogen sulphide and much else. See Chapter 4, page 42, for how to get rid of UFG with the PK diet, vitamin C 5 g daily and Lugol's iodine 15 % 3 drops at night

What	Why and How
Tap water	Much tap water contains, for example, chlorine and fluoride.[1] Cleanse tap water with activated charcoal. I recommend a large glass Kilner jar with a tap at the bottom and some sticks of activated charcoal. Fill from the tap at night and by the morning you will have delicious water
Prescription drugs	The vast majority suppress symptoms. Address the underlying cause then tail them off (see our book *Ecological Medicine*)
Vaccines	All contain toxic adjuvants to stimulate the immune system. Some contain mercury and many contain aluminium adjuvants in nano-particle size; this is especially pernicious[2]
Household cleaning agents, cosmetics, perfumes and other such volatile organic compounds (VOCs)	If you can smell it, then it is in your brain. Do not put anything on your skin that you are not prepared to eat… except pure soap
Dental amalgam, dental metals, piercings	Mercury, nickel, silver, tin, cadmium, lead, antimony. See my website for the toxicity of mercury[3]
Seafood	This is all contaminated with toxic metals, especially mercury, and pesticides, especially the organochlorines, and probably radioactivity[4]
Electromagnetic pollution	Especially 5G, wifi, mobile and cordless phones (see my website[5])
Air pollution: ozone, particulate matter, sulphur dioxide, nitrogen dioxide, carbon monoxide and lead	Do your best to avoid these. Consider air filtration system
Tattoos and hair dyes	Dyes are one of the commonest blockers found on mitochondrial translocator proteins. Tattoos contain phthlates (one of the Environmental Working Group's 'Dirty Dozen'[7]), toxic metals and hydrocarbons[7, 8]
Pesticides in food, gardens, and for insect control generally	Glyphosate is currently the greatest threat. It has never been more important to eat organic food. I would far rather my PBs (see page xvi) spent precious resources on food than clinical tests which do not change management[9]

Table 14.1 *Cont'd*

What	Why and How
Mycotoxins from water-damaged buildings and cellars and from fungal infection of the airways and gut	The best way to diagnose fungal driven pathology is to go for a holiday in an environment where the humidity is less than 40% - either a hot dry climate, cold dry, above 3000 ft (1000 m) or right on the coast where winds are on-shore (fungi cannot grow on/in salt water)
Silicone e.g. breast implants, testicular implants, mesh for hernia repair, tubes and pipes, body contouring. Contraceptive implant	Silicone is soft and 'outgases' from the day implants are inserted. The immune system recognises it as a foreigner and attacks it, but silicone is a plastic and cannot be broken down in the body. The attack cannot 'kill' silicone, but much damage ensues from friendly fire[10]
Surgical metals	Sometimes these are essential. The key to safe surgery is to do all one can to prevent inflammation, then use single, low-allergy-potential metals. Avoid mixed metals or you get a battery effect
Microplastics	We are all polluted with microplastics. They pose a risk to humans in three different ways: physical, chemical and as a host for other microorganisms to gather and breed on.[11] Avoid using plastics (plates, cups, wrappings) and use paper or wood alternatives Wear natural fibres

Additional notes to support Table 14.1

Fluoride in water: In 2014, authors Stephen Peckham and Niyi Awofeso concluded that: 'Fluoride has modest benefit in terms of reduction of dental caries but significant costs in relation to cognitive impairment, hypothyroidism, dental and skeletal fluorosis, enzyme and electrolyte derangement, and uterine cancer.'[1] If you are in the UK, you can see whether your water is fluoridated here: www.uk-water-filters.co.uk/pages/areas-with-fluoride-added-to-drinking-and-tap-water

Vaccinations: The authors of a 2013 paper on nanoparticles for vaccine celivery, including Diane Williamson from the UK Government's Defence

Science and Technology Laboratory at Porton Down, concluded that: 'Since NPs (nanoparticles) have a relatively short history in medicine they do not have a longstanding safety profile in human use. It is therefore essential that further research is carried out in NP toxicity to fully address these questions if they are to be accepted as an alternative method for the delivery of novel vaccines and are licensed more widely for human use.' And '…it is also worth noting their potential drawbacks, particularly those associated with cytotoxicity.' (Cytotoxicity = damage to cells.)[2]

Seafood: To give just one example, authors Guo et al in 2007 concluded that seafood was highly contaminated with dichlorodiphenyltrichloroethane (DDT) and that this might pose a human health threat both to local coastal populations and to consumers of seafood far and wide. In addition, the authors found that components of organochlorine pesticides (OCP), also found in seafood, conferred a lifetime cancer risk, in this case especially to local coastal populations, who often consume more seafood than other populations.[4]

Tattoos: A 2022 study concluded that, amongst other things, the ingredients of tattoo inks include polycyclic aromatic hydrocarbons (PAHs), heavy metals (cadmium, lead, mercury, antimony, beryllium and arsenic) and primary aromatic amines (PAAs), and that these could pose toxicological carcinogenic risks to human health.[7] A 2011 paper had looked at phthalates specifically in black tattoo inks.[7]

Glyphosate: A common commercial name for glyphosate, used as a weedkiller, is Roundup. In 2015, Robin Mesnage and colleagues concluded that: 'Our results suggest that chronic exposure to a GBH in an established laboratory animal toxicity model system at an ultra-low, environmental dose can result in liver and kidney damage with potential significant health implications for animal and human populations.'[9]

Detox

We then need to detox. The mechanisms by which we get rid of toxins involve micronutrients.

Micronutrients

Good nutrition is highly protective against toxic stress. All the nutritional interventions that you have in place with the Groundhog regimes (see Appendix 1) help to get rid of toxins AND mitigate their toxicity.

Look at thalidomide and what its selective toxic effects show up. This drug was prescribed to women in pregnancy as a 'pregnancy-safe hypnotic' (that is, a 'sleeping pill') but only caused serious birth defects if taken during early pregnancy. This drug was tested in rats and no offspring were abnormal. This was a mystery to researchers, until someone had the bright idea of putting the rats onto nutritionally depleted diets. Then the baby rats developed the foetal abnormality of phocomelia (horribly dubbed 'flipper limbs') that was the problem occurring in humans. It was a combination of toxic stress (the drug) *and* nutritional deficiency at a critical stage of foetal development which caused the problem to become apparent.

How to reduce the body's load of VOCs and pesticides using heating regimes

Many toxic chemicals are dumped in fat – this includes fat in the brain, bone marrow and, of course, all membranes. They do not get into the bloodstream for the liver to get rid. This is where heating regimes are so helpful because they mobilise chemicals from these tissues. The idea of heating regimes is to heat up subcutaneous fat and literally boil off these toxins. They migrate through the skin onto the surface where they dissolve in the fatty lipid layer that covers the skin, whence* they can be washed off. It is not essential to sweat for these regimes to be effective but the washing off is as important as the heat. If not washed off the toxins will simply be reabsorbed.

Some toxins will mobilise into the bloodsteam and that may cause acute poisoning, so it is important to start regimes with low heats and short times and build up slowly.

I have collected data from over 30 patients who have undergone tests of toxicity both before and after these heating regimes. The tests have been chosen for particular situations but include fat biopsies, translocator protein studies and DNA adducts. The tests prove to my satisfaction that heating regimes are effective. These heating regimes include:

- sauna: traditional and far infrared (FIR)
- Epsom Salt hot baths.

I would expect sunbathing and exercise to be just as effective. Indeed, similar research was conducted by Dr William Rea in America and he used similar regimes of massage, gentle exercise, sauna-ing and showering to achieve very similar biochemical results.[12] Dr Rea concluded that 63% of a cohort of 210 patients had reduced levels of toxic chemicals after treatment and that this led to clinical improvements in 31% of those with autonomic nervous system disorders.

My experience, roughly speaking, is that 50 episodes will halve the body load. One would expect chemicals to come out exponentially, so one never gets to zero, but one ends up in some sort of equilibrium with the environment which is as low as reasonably possible. Indeed, because we live in such a toxic world, I think we should all be doing some sort of heating regime at least once a week. My personal preference is for Epsom salt baths.

[*]**Linguistic note:** 'Hence', 'thence' and 'whence' are examples of a legacy (Latin) 'ablative' case, still in use in the English language. The ablative case is used to express motion away from something, among other uses. So, we have:
Hence – from here
Thence – from there
Whence – from where.

In much less common usage, and so sometimes referred to as 'fossil words', are the locative cases – in Latin, the locative denotes 'place where something is or occurs'. So, we have:
Hither – to here, to this place
Thither – to there, to that place
Whither – to where, to which place.

In the film, *The Life of Brian*, John Cleese's Roman Centurion becomes very angry with Graham Chapman's 'Brian', who is daubing the anti-Roman graffito, 'Romans go home', and dares to get the locative case wrong! See https://www.youtube.com/watch?v=IIAdHEwiAy8

Indeed, it is my view that because we live in such a toxic world we should not wait until we become ill, we should be using detox regimes on a regular basis and those regimes, in my opinion, should include heating regimes. Take advantage of what is available locally to detox your system on a weekly basis. For those people lucky enough to live in a hot climate, an hour of sunbathing followed by a dip in the sea is ideal. The Ancients knew the benefits of sunbathing and even had a verb for it – *apricari* (to bask in the sunshine). This gives us one of the great unused words in the English language – to apricate, meaning to bask in the sunshine.

We English relish hot baths, and the effect of detoxification is further enhanced by adding Epsom salts into the bath. The idea here is that not only are the toxins pulled out by the heat but magnesium and sulphate pass through the skin into the body – both magnesium and sulphate are essential co-factors to allow detoxification. This was established in a lovely study by Dr Rosemary Waring at Birmingham University (see https://en.wikipedia.org/wiki/Rosemary_Waring) who showed that both magnesium and sulphate levels in the blood increased markedly following such hot baths, as did the excretion of magnesium sulphate in the urine. Her formula was for 500 g Epsom salts in 15 gallons of water. We English also love to mix our metric and imperial measurements! OK, OK… 15 gallons is 68 litres.[13] Here in UK you can get a delivery of kilograms of magnesium sulphate from www.epsomsalts.co.uk. If you do not possess a bath, you can purchase a 'shower bath' for a good soaking.

For countries with a tradition of sauna-ing, this is another excellent method of pulling out toxins through the skin. Indeed, I recall a case of one family who were all poisoned by organophosphate and had high levels in their fat biopsies. They decided to take themselves off for a three-week holiday in Eastern Europe at a lovely hotel which offered regular massage, sauna-ing, hot springs and mineral bath treatments. They all cycled from one treatment to the next. The results were little short of astonishing – after three weeks of treatment their toxic load of organophosphates had reduced substantially, almost to background levels.

Some people feel terrible following heating regimes as toxins are mobilised into the bloodstream (see Appendix 2: DDD reactions). It may be that such reactions are a useful clinical measure of one's combined toxic and infectious load. Indeed, one can do a urine test for toxins, but this is pricey. Curiosity is an expensive hobby! This clinical test (i.e. do you have a detox reaction) is a useful guide to toxicity. Should detox reactions occur, reduce the time, heat and frequency to that which is bearable. With time this will improve.

How to reduce the body's load of toxic metals using detox tools

Heating regimes do not get rid of toxic metals. If there is a suspicion of toxic metal exposure, then tests are helpful to measure the load and monitor response to treatment. Simple hair analysis or urine tests can produce false negatives. For a reliable result we need to measure levels following a dose of chelating DMSA (that's 2,3-demercapto-succinic acid, for the boffins). For this test, empty the bladder, take DMSA 15 mg per kg of body weight, collect urine for six hours, then send a sample off to the lab (see Useful resources, page 303. Look for Comprehensive Urine Element Profile at either www.gdx.net or https://smartnutrition.co.uk). DMSA will also grab friendly minerals such as copper, zinc, chromium, manganese and selenium – so expect to see high levels of these.

If toxins are high, then DMSA can also be used to detox. Because DMSA also chelates friendly minerals, it should be taken only once a week and one should not take friendly mineral supplements on one's 'DMSA day', but then take good doses of friendly minerals on the other days to rescue the situation for the other six days of the week. My experience is that most poisoned patients need at least 12 weeks of DMSA, after which the test can be repeated. This gives us two points on the graph and an idea of how much more, if any, chelation is required to reduce the body load to an acceptable level. One can never get the body load to zero – all one can do is establish a reasonable equilibrium with the external environment.

If DMSA is not tolerated (this is rare), then there are other ways to treat toxic metals. All the supplements listed in Table 14.2 are of proven effectiveness. In practice I suggest putting in place as many of these as are tolerable and/or affordable.

Table 14.2: Supplements which help detox. (As you can see, many are part of Groundhog regimes)

Supplement	Mechanism	Maximum dose
Zinc, selenium and magnesium	Displace toxic metals from binding sites in the body…	Zinc 50 mg, selenium 500 mcg Magnesium 300 mg: no oral maximum dose but diarrhoea if too much
Glutathione	…so the toxic metals can be picked up by glutathione and excreted	No maximum dose, but 250-500 mg is usual
Vitamin C to bowel tolerance	Vital antioxidant – the final repository of free radicals	The dose is key, and everyone is different
	Binds to toxic metals so they can be excreted in urine	Vitamin C also pulls out friendly minerals, so it is vital to take Sunshine salt to replace the 'lost' 'good' minerals
Iodine	Binds to toxic metals so they can be excreted in urine	Lugol's iodine 15% 2-4 drops daily (take at night away from vitamin C)
High-fat diet. Several dessertspoons of organic hemp oil	'Washes out' the polluted fats in the body and replaces them with clean fats. Phospholipids can be given intravenously (IV) to good effect	Oral fats and oils probably work as well as IV but it takes much longer
Vitamin B12 and correcting homocysteine	Improves the methylation cycle – sticking a methyl group onto toxins renders them water-soluble so they are peed out	B12 is extremely safe. Take at least 5 mg sublingually daily. Consider B12 injections
	If homocysteine is low, then correct with…	
You can test homocysteine easily on a DIY blood test (see Useful resources, page 303)	Methyl B12 as above, methyl B6 (pyridoxal 5 phosphate) 50 mg and methyl tetrahydrofolate 800 mcg daily	
Adsorbant clays†	See below	

Monitoring progress

Whichever technique is used, you need to retest to make sure it is working. If not, consider the possibility of unrecognised ongoing exposure. For example:

1. Is the mercury coming from incomplete amalgam removal?
2. Or fish in the diet?

How to reduce the load of mycotoxins

First, identify the source of production, which may be outside or inside the body. Chapter 4 looks at mycotoxins with a source inside the body; the fermenting gut produces fungal mycotoxins. Treat this problem with PK diet, vitamin C and Lugol's Iodine.

Other sources include chronic fungal sinusitis, chronic fungal chest infection (start with iodine salt pipe) and chronic perineal infection (make your own iodine oil – 10 parts coconut oil mixed with one part Lugol's Iodine).

The main source outside the body is water-damaged buildings.

Then use clays to mop up mycotoxins from the gut – see next.

Adsorbant clays to get rid of toxic metals and mycotoxins

Many fat-soluble toxins, such as VOCs and pesticides, are excreted in the fatty bile salts produced by the liver, only to be reabsorbed lower down in the intestine. This is called the enterohepatic circulation. However, clays will adsorb such toxins so they can be excreted in faeces. This is a benign way to remove toxins since they are not mobilised into the bloodstream and so do not cause detox reactions. Clays will also remove

[†]**Spelling footnote:**This is not a typo. A**d**sorption and a**b**sorption mean quite different things. Absorption is where a liquid is soaked up into something like a sponge, cloth or filter paper. The liquid is completely absorbed into the absorbent material. Adsorption refers to individual molecules, atoms or ions gathering on surfaces.

friendly minerals. Thus, I suggest taking the away from food and supplements, e.g. last thing at night. There are many clays with good potential, but I tend to use inexpensive diatomaceous earth or food clay, 3 g (a heaped teaspoonful), stirred into water and swallowed. This does not taste too bad – elephants seek out and love river clay and I am very happy to be compared to an elephant!‡

Improve energy delivery mechanisms

The liver uses 27% of all the energy generated by the body and much of this is consumed by detox enzymes. The kidneys demand constant energy delivery; they do not tolerate anything less. Improving energy delivery also improves detox.

‡**Historical note:** 'Geophagia' is the word used to describe the deliberate consumption of earth, soil or clay. It has been widely regarded as a psychiatric disease. Indeed, the standard reference guide for psychiatrists—the fourth edition of the *Diagnostic and Statistical Manual for Mental Disorders (DSM-IV)* — classifies geophagia as a subtype of pica, an eating disorder in which people consume things that are not food, such as cigarette ash. However, studies of animals and human cultures suggest that geophagia is not necessarily a madness. It is prevalent in more than 200 species of animals, including parrots, deer, elephants, bats, rabbits, baboons, gorillas and chimpanzees. It is also well documented in humans, with Pliny (Gaius Plinius Secundus, 23 – 79 AD) describing the popularity of *alica*, a porridge-like cereal that contained red clay: 'Used as a drug it has a soothing effect... as a remedy for ulcers in the humid part of the body such as the mouth or anus.'[14] Maybe this is another example of the Ancients not knowing why this practice worked but forging ahead anyway, on the strength of the clinical results.

Summary

- Exposure to toxic metals, pesticides, VOCs, prescription drugs, mycotoxins etc, is bad for you.
- Try to avoid exposure.
- Then get rid of these by:
  - Taking my Groundhog micronutrient packages.
  - For VOCs and pesticides by using heating regimes.
  - For heavy metals by using the detox tools as above – i.e. supplements, high-fat diet, and adsorbant clays.
  - For endogenous mycotoxins, use PK diet, vitamin C and Lugol's iodine and for exogenous mycotoxins, use adsorbant clays.
- Improve energy delivery mechanisms, as this will give the liver the energy to deal with all detoxifications.

Chapter 15

The general approach to treating chronic infection

Even when we do not know what the microbes are there is much we can do to treat chronic infection.

Reduce the infectious load

All chronic infection starts with an acute infection. When it dates from such and is characterised by fatigue and inflammation, we call this ME.

Acute infection can be dealt with in two ways. One is to get rid of it completely and acquire natural immunity so it is never a problem again (except for overwhelming numbers). The second way is to reduce the numbers of microbes in the body to such a level that they no longer constitute a threat. This is how we deal with the herpes viruses (all of which subsequently infect us for life). All acute infection should be treated with Groundhog Acute (Appendix 1). However, by the time people come to see me they usually have a chronic infection.

We know that pretty much all pathology has an infectious driver. There is much more detail in our book *The Infection Game* but the basics are:

- Dementia may be driven by herpes viruses, HIV or Lyme.[1, 2, 3]
- Arterial disease may be driven by Covid-19,[4] or the gram-negative bacteria of gum disease.[5]
- Cancer may be driven by *Helicobacter pylori*, Epstein Barr virus, human papilloma virus and more.[6]

The question we need to ask is why some people get these diseases but others do not. The answer is… it is all about good immunity. We need good immune function to keep the numbers of microbes as low as is possible.

We all love simple solutions to problems. Sir Isaac Newton (English mathematician, 25 December 1642 – 20 March 1726/27) was no exception when he said: 'Truth is ever to be found in the simplicity, and not in the multiplicity and confusion of things.' But Newton was dealing with the motion of the planets and other such matters – easier things to understand than the human body, a fact which he himself admitted, when he uttered the memorable words: 'I can calculate the motion of heavenly bodies, but not the madness of people.'

My patients with ME want to be told that their symptoms are caused by EBV and can be got rid of with valaciclovir, or they have Lyme which can be got rid of with antibiotics or they have fungal infection to be abolished with anti-fungals. This is rarely the case. Once you have one microbe in the body that is winning the arms race, immunity is suppressed, and others move in. These are called 'co-infections'. I suspect that the vast majority of people with disease have multiple infections and the immune system is fighting on all fronts to deal with these. Multiple infections cause inflammation and, because the immune system needs much energy to fight, fatigue. This gives us the clinical picture of ME (myalgic-encephalitis). These people are losing the arms race.

The treatment of ME and any disease associated with chronic infection

To tackle chronic infection, first we need to apply everything in the preceding chapters. For many, that is all that is necessary. Secondly, we put in place all possible interventions to reduce the numbers of microbes. This is what this chapter and the next two are about. In order:

1. Herbal antimicrobials (see next).
2. DMSO to destroy biofilms and improve microcirculation (Chapter 16).
3. Methylene blue (Chapter 17).
4. Light therapy (Chapter 18).

Herbal antimicrobials

Plants and fungi have been similarly involved in the arms race even longer than mammals. They too are survivors and have evolved equally intelligent and effective strategies to fight off microbial attack. We can jump on their bandwagon by eating them. There is a massive scientific literature detailing the benefits of plants and fungi in the fight against infectious disease. A definitive guide for those who wish to study this in greater detail is *Herbal Medicine 2nd Edition*, edited by Iris F F Benzie and Sissi Wachtel-Galor.[7]

Some work by killing microbes directly, but many of the beneficial effects result from impacts on the immune system. These can form an important part of improving the defences.

The starting point is to regularly consume any herb, spice or mushroom that you can get your hands on, in large amounts. Initially, at least, I do not think it matters much which you go for, because they all have antimicrobial benefits all being modern-day survivors. However, I am greatly influenced by taste, availability and, being naturally mean, cost. I am fortunate to have a garden with a variety of herbs which are a joy to collect and consume. Many do not even get into the kitchen – I am currently scoffing parsley, rocket and wild garlic. My favourite hill grows parasols and horse mushrooms in season. My top-of-the-pops herbs for dishes I detail in our book *Paleo-Ketogenic: The Why and the How*, and include garlic, black pepper, ginger, rosemary, mint and thyme. I love Indian dishes with turmeric, cardamom, coriander and cummin. We are so fortunate to live in a world with access to all these delights.

Much of the herbology I have learned from the books of Stephen Buhner, medical herbalist. Sadly, Stephen Buhner died on 8th December 2022, and was buried in his beloved forest. You can read an obituary here: https://planetthrive.com/2022/12/rip-stephen-buhner/ He had a similarly irreverent, and refreshing, view of orthodoxy. He liked to give his patients the knowledge and the tools of the trade so they could sort themselves out.

Buhner wrote several books, all a delight to read, with essential and useful practical clinical information. However, I suspect the abundance of information he supplied may make it difficult for the fatigued, foggy-brained, sick patient to know where to start. For details of the biology, pharmacology, cultivation, preparation, variety of uses and clinical applications, you must read his books. I shall confine myself to the bare minimum of what you need to know to get started.

Many herbs multitask, so I have picked out four herbs which improve the ‘defences’ (that is, support the immune system) and therefore have application in each and every infectious disease – namely, astragalus, cordyceps, rhodiola and Chinese skullcap. They have some additional antimicrobial actions as well as being immune-supportive. All have the potential to help in fatigue syndromes because of a multiplicity of effects, improving mitochondrial function (and therefore immune function) and reducing any infectious load.

These herbs further qualify for inclusion because they are all extremely safe, remarkably free from side effects and relatively inexpensive. These are the real super foods. Astragalus and cordyceps should be included in one’s regular diet as a food rather than as a medicine.

Table 15.1: Herbal antimicrobials

Herb	Effects	Dose	Notes
Astragalus (a legume)	Assists with delivery of energy and raw materials to foot soldiers and officers. Provides ammunition. Improves communication to prevent friendly fire. Helps to mop up the damage which inevitably results in killing zones. Directly toxic to many viruses (flu, HHV1, CMV, Hep B and others) Antibacterial (Staph, Strep, E coli, Lyme and others) Antifungal (candida) Also anti-covid[8]	Whole root powder 15-60 g per day taken in three separate doses. Start with a low dose and build up. As with all antimicrobials in chronic infection, one can get a die-off or Herxheimer reaction.[*] In this event, reduce the dose a little, wait for symptoms to settle, then retry a higher dose	The sliced root in soup and stews is delicious. It also makes a good tea; it has a slightly sweet taste. It can be chewed raw as a chewing gum alternative
Cordyceps[†] (a fungus)	Improves energy delivery from mitochondria. Assists with delivery of energy and raw materials to foot soldiers and officers. Provides ammunition . Improves communication to prevent friendly fire. Helps to mop up the damage which inevitably results in killing zones. Antiviral (against 'flu, HHV1, HIV, Hep B) Antibacterial (TB, Staph, Strep) Anti-fungal (candida) Kills mycoplasma Also anti-covid[9]	Whole fungus 3-9 g per day. Up to 50 g in acute infection. NB: May lower blood sugar so diabetics on medication must be aware – more reason to get PK-adapted (see Chapter 2) before you start	This makes a superb treat: • Melt together equal weights of cocoa fat, coconut oil and cordyceps powder. • Tip some goji berries into paper cup cake moulds and cover with the melted mix. • Store in, and eat directly from, the fridge

Herb	Effects	Dose	Notes
Rhodiola (looks like a sedum (stonecrop))	Especially used for neuroprotection. Improves energy delivery from mitochondria. Assists with delivery of energy and raw materials to foot soldiers and officers. Provides ammunition. Improves communication to prevent friendly fire. Helps to mop up the damage which inevitably results in killing zones. Antiviral (against 'flu, Hep C, Coxsackie B) Antibacterial (against Staph, TB) Also anti-covid[10]	Use the whole herb in capsules twice daily, up to 1000 mg per day NB: Some people feel a bit jittery with rhodiola. I suspect this is due to low blood sugar – all the more reason to get PK-adapted!	1 tsp leaves with boiling water poured over make a good tea
Chinese skullcap	Especially good for killing EBV and herpes viruses; these are common drivers of ME. Remarkably safe herb. It kills viruses in many ways, including inhibiting neuraminidase and haemaglutinin, inhibiting viral replication, inhibiting viral entry into host cells, reducing cytokine cascades and being directly toxic to virus. Also anti-covid[11]	Buhner recommends using the root as a powder 1-3 g taken three times daily	

Remember with all the herbs in Table 15.1, and indeed any new intervention, start with a low dose and build up slowly.

[*]**Note:** A Herxheimer reaction can be a reaction to endotoxin-like products released by the death of harmful micro-organisms within the body. The contents of 'burst' microbial cells are released into the body and this has a temporary toxic effect until such toxins can be cleared out of the system; it can also be an allergy-like reaction (see Appendix 2, page 247).

[†]**Note:** For fans of *The Last of Us*, this is most definitely NOT the cordyceps of the 'Cordyceps Brain Infection' of that TV series.[12]

DMSO (dimethyl sulphoxide)

The next step is to use DMSO, for which see Chapter 16.

Microbes make themselves at home in the body with biofilm. This creates a protective layer so they can hide from the immune system. The example of biofilm that we all know about is dental plaque, produced by the tooth-rotting bacterium *Streptococcus mutans*. DMSO may dissolve biofilm. A 2017 study by Yahaya and colleagues concluded that DMSO inhibited many biological pathways and in so doing, this reduced the development of biofilm.[13]

Improve microcirculation

THEN you improve the microcirculation, so the white cells of the immune system contact the microbes to kill 'em. DMSO reduces the friction so blood flow is enhanced. (It does this through its impact on the fourth phase of water – see Chapter 5.) As an example, in their 1989 study, Murav'ev and colleagues concluded that DMSO represented a therapeutic intervention for rheumatic diseases due its ability to regularise the formation of fibrin and its balancing action on microcirculation.[14]

Methylene blue (MB)

THEN you should use methylene blue, for which please turn to Chapter 17. This is a broad-spectrum antimicrobial.

Light therapy

FINALLY, we should supercharge all the interventions above with light, for which please go to Chapter 18. Red light and near infrared activate MB. Far infrared further reduces the numbers of microbes and improves energy delivery mechanisms among its multiple benefits.[15] As with all treatments, start with a low dose (in terms of temperature and time of exposure) and build up gradually. This is called photodynamic therapy.[16]

Summary

- Most major pathologies, including CFS, ME and LC, are driven by chronic infections.
- The reason that some people develop these pathologies and others don't, is the difference having a good immune system makes.
- We can help the immune system and reduce the infectious load with:
    - Herbals – astragalus, cordyceps, rhodiola and Chinese skullcap.
    - DMSO – see Chapter 16.
    - Methylene blue – see Chapter 17.
    - And we can supercharge all of these with light – see Chapter 18.

Chapter 16

Dimethylsulphoxide (DMSO) – an antimicrobial tool

DMS (dimethylsulphide*) is produced by marine phytoplankton and oxidised to DMSO† in the atmosphere. It is normally present in the human body and many foods (fruit, vegetables and grain). It probably plays a major role in the natural transfer of sulphur of biological origin, according to a 1987 paper in the prestigious journal *Nature* of which James Lovelock† (originator of Gaia theory) was a co-author.[1] This makes DMSO an early evolutionary player for all things sulphur related.

***Historical note:** Dimethylsulphoxide was first synthesised in 1866 by the Russian scientist Alexander Zaytsev. Alexander had an obtuse route into the study of chemistry. He was the son of a tea and sugar merchant who wanted him also to be a merchant. However, an uncle persuaded him to enrol at the University of Kazan to study economics. At this time, Russia was experimenting with the cameral system, meaning that every student graduating in law and economics from a Russian university had to take two years of chemistry. Thus, after many more twists and turns, we end up with DMSO, and also Zaytsev's rule (interested readers can look up this fine piece of empirical chemistry).

†**Note from Craig:** James Lovelock is one of my heroes. A man before his time, highly individual, shunned by conventional scientists, and finally proven right on all of his predictions. Now why is it that I like Sarah so much?! Oh, and James Lovelock saved the world by inventing the electron capture detector in his 'work' shed, at the bottom of his back garden. It was this device that proved the persistence of chlorofluorocarbons (CFCs) in the atmosphere and their role in ozone depletion, leading to the banning of CFC products. Lovelock died on his 103rd birthday on 26 July 2022. Interested readers are urged to watch the BBC Documentary *Beautiful Minds* on James Lovelock – it is about an hour long: www.youtube.com/watch?v=QqwZJDEZ9Ng

Sulphate is a much forgotten molecule in the body. It binds to many molecules to allow them to circulate safely in the bloodstream before being released at their target site. This includes cholesterol. (Cholesterol should circulate as cholesterol sulphate; if one is sulphate deficient then it circulates in the form of LDL and so high LDL may be symptomatic of sulphate deficiency and is not per se 'unfriendly').

I have been using DMSO for decades as a delivery molecule for transdermal magnesium. However, it has wonderful properties in its own right and, being so safe, this gives it a multiplicity of uses.

Table 16.1: The physical and chemical properties of DMSO

DMSO properties	What this means	Use
It is a small molecule with a similar shape and polarity to water	Dissolves readily in water and passes through all tissues of the body	It is well absorbed through the skin and can be applied to skin to treat any condition anywhere in the body
		Sprayed on the skin it is rapidly absorbed together with any minerals, magnesium, vitamins B12, D or C that you care to mix with it. You can see my transdermal preparations on my website (see Useful resources page 303)
It improves the quality of the fourth phase of water ('exclusion zone water' or 'gel water').[2] This reduces the friction between all surfaces. This effect is amplified by far infrared light	This would explain its known action as an anti-inflammatory. Useful for any autoimmune condition	Can be used to treat any condition associated with inflammation – e.g. for bursitis, tendonitis, muscle tears[3]

Table 16.1 *Cont'd*

DMSO properties	What this means	Use
	An anticoagulant	Can be used to treat any condition associated with clotting. Intravenous DMSO has been used to dissolve blood clots and so reverse strokes and heart attacks
	Improves blood supply by reducing the friction between blood cells and blood vessel walls	Can be used to treat any condition associated with poor blood supply, e.g. angina, poor circulation
	Analgesic effect	Can be used to treat any condition that is painful! Used in migraine topically (massage onto the scalp) and by mouth
It is a close relative of important sulphur compounds in the body and may be converted into glucosamine, MSM, chondroitin, alpha lipoic acid, allicin (from garlic), N-acetyl cysteine, SAME (S-adenosylmethionine) and glutathione and so is the raw material of connective tissue	Building blocks of skin, tendons, membranes, muscles	Accelerates healing and repair. Use for any acute injury, painful area, acute arthritis
Essential for detoxification	Gets rid of toxic metals and other such toxins. Sulphur binds with toxic heavy metals (mercury, lead, aluminium, cadmium, arsenic, nickel) and eliminates them via urination, defaecation and sweating	To detoxify the body. This effect is so powerful that it may trigger a detox reaction (see Appendix 2)
Essential for methylation	We need methylation to read DNA and make proteins	For healing and repair

DMSO properties	What this means	Use
In low doses it is an antioxidant	Slows degeneration. Protects mitochondria. Helps to prevent cancer. Protects against radiation	This gives DMSO application for almost any condition of the human body[4]
In high doses (and an acid environment) it is a pro-oxidant It may dissolve biofilm	So is antiviral, antibacterial and antifungal	Again, this effect is so powerful that it may trigger a die-off or Herxheimer reaction (see Appendix 2)
It is a universal solvent	To soften connective tissue or scar tissue	Scleroderma Old scars or injuries To accelerate healing and repair

The mechanisms by which DMSO is so helpful give us its clinical application. It has around 40 pharmacological properties that may be beneficial in the prevention, relief or reversal of numerous diseases.[5]

Table 16.2: The clinical uses of DMSO

Mechanisms of action	So, it can be used for:	Clinical pictures such as:	By mouth	By skin – apply to affected area
DMSO is an antioxidant – it readily donates electrons and this makes it good at scavenging free radicals	Any condition associated with inflammation. Inflammation is characterised by pain	Interstitial cystitis (DMSO it has an FDA licence to treat this[6]	Yes	Yes
Local anaesthetic effect	Useful as a pain reliever. For any painful joint or muscle. This effect will be enhanced by adding magnesium	Arthritis Fibromyalgia Headaches and migraine Tic doloureaux Complex regional pain syndrome[6]	Yes	Yes With magnesium

Table 16.2 *Cont'd*

Mechanisms of action	So, it can be used for:	Clinical pictures such as:	By mouth	By skin – apply to affected area
		Any painful site e.g. shingles, chicken pox Dental pain		Yes
	Research suggests that applying DMSO 50% to the skin improves pain in people with complex regional pain syndrome[7]			Yes
	To heal and repair tissue damage. Any such damage anywhere in the body can be accessed by DMSO because it easily passes through all body tissues	Sprains, strains, bursitis, tendonitis, frozen shoulder, keloids, scars	Yes	Yes
It improves blood supply. (I suspect this is because it promotes the fourth phase of water)	Any condition associated with poor blood supply or blood clotting	DMSO has been used to treat angina, heart failure, intermittent claudication, dementia	Yes	
	Cholesterol should be carried in blood as the soluble cholesterol sulphate – when there is sulphur deficiency we see a high level of LDL cholesterol (which is not 'unfriendly').	Ditto	Yes	

Mechanisms of action	**So, it can be used for:**	**Clinical pictures such as:**	**By mouth**	**By skin – apply to affected area**
Improves mitochondrial function (Again because of its effects on the fourth phase of water)	AGAIN Any condition associated with poor energy delivery mechanisms	Chronic fatigue syndrome	Yes	Yes
A source of sulphur and so good for detoxing heavy metals	Arteriosclerosis	AGAIN DMSO has been used to treat angina, heart failure, intermittent claudication, dementia	Yes	
Dissolves biofilm	Good for any skin infection	Acne, cold sores Fungal infections: tinea, jock itch, ring worm, rosacea		Paint on a 50% solution to which a few drops of Lugol's 15% iodine has been added
Dissolves viral lipid coat	Cold sores, chicken pox or shingles Herpes viruses Coronavirus	Chronic infections	Yes	Paint on a 50% solution 3 times daily with iodine as above
	Upper fermenting gut (of proven benefit for *Helicobacter pylori*)	Indigestion, burping, bloating, pain	Yes	
Kills bacteria in the mouth	The fermenting mouth	Gum disease, tooth decay		Rinse the mouth with a 50% solution

Table 16.2 *Cont'd*

Mechanisms of action	So, it can be used for:	Clinical pictures such as:	By mouth	By skin – apply to affected area
and sinuses		Respiratory infections, especially sinusitis	Yes	Can be used in a nebuliser with a few drops of Lugol's iodine 15%
DMSO dissolves amyloid	May be indicated for prion disorders[8]	These include Alzheimer's disease and Parkinson's disease (DMSO passes through the blood-brain barrier)	Yes	
Dissolves stones	Dissolves stones[9]	Kidney stones and gallstones	Yes	
Is mildly anti-cholinesterase – increases acetyl choline	Helpful for depression and anxiety		Yes	
Essential raw material for healing and repair	Early research suggests that applying DMSO to the skin might help the skin heal after surgery.		Yes	Yes
All the above	Diseases of the eye	Especially macular degeneration, cataracts, glaucoma	Yes	Yes – 2 drops of 2.5% DMSO into each eye
				Or rub the eyelids with 40% solution
	Leaky gut		Yes	

Mechanisms of action	So, it can be used for:	Clinical pictures such as:	By mouth	By skin – apply to affected area
	Any condition associated with poor circulation such as venous ulcers			Yes
		Skin anti-ageing		With coconut oil and vitamin C

How to use DMSO

Do all else detailed in this book first. Then I can see this is going to become another favourite multi-tasking tool.

How to purchase DMSO

It must be as very pure 99.9% source, and should be in glass bottles (or failing that, resistant plastic). See my website as one possible source (Useful resources, page 303).

At a concentration of 99.9%, DMSO goes solid below 18ºC. Should this happen, warm it up by placing the bottle of DMSO in warm water or keep it in a warm room. This does not affect its qualities in any way.

How to take DMSO

By mouth: You can consume DMSO without dilution. When mixed with water it generates heat so this may give you a warm sensation in your mouth. Some people prefer to dilute it in a small glass of water. Take this twice per day. It is very safe. I suggest 10-20 ml DMSO daily

By skin: DMSO passes through the skin like a knife through butter. This means that any contaminants on the skin (cosmetics, chemicals, dirt) will be washed into the body. Therefore, ONLY APPLY DMSO TO THE SKIN WHEN IT IS ABSOLUTELY CLEAN. Similarly, DMSO will affect tattoos and flush the metals of piercings into the body. Therefore, do NOT apply DMSO to tattoos or around jewellery. It can be used as a 20% solution (my transdermal sprays are 20%) or make a 50% solution (half parts water, half DMSO). More concentrated solutions may cause local heat and redness. Apply up to four times per day.

Combined with other ingredients: My transdermal preparations (see Useful resources, page 303) are good for enhancing the absorption of a range of nutrients. These contain 20% DMSO.

Troubleshooting

This is mostly repetition but of the utmost importance:

- Do not use DMSO on skin at concentrations greater than 50% or it may cause itching, redness and possibly dryness of the skin.
- Any other side effects, such as stomach upset, headaches, dizziness, and sedation, are very likely related to detoxification reactions prompted by the DMSO. I suspect these are largely a problem where there is an upper fermenting gut (see page 40), so make sure you have Groundhog Chronic (page 240) in place.
- Only purified and properly diluted DMSO should be used. When you dilute a pure DMSO solution, always do so in spring water.
- When it is applied to skin, make sure the skin and applying hand are thoroughly cleaned and rinsed before application. This is of utmost importance as DMSO's properties allow contaminants to be absorbed through the skin and transported into the bloodstream. DMSO is known to be one of the least toxic substances in biology.[10] Any side effects would come from potential contaminants or the intake of concomitant drugs that DMSO will carry into the body or a detox/die-off reaction.
- DMSO, and any substance dissolved in it, will penetrate the skin, the blood-brain barrier and other parts of the body very fast.
- DMSO increases the effects of drugs like blood thinners, steroids, heart medicines, sedatives, etc.
- Acetone or acid contamination of DMSO can lead to serious medical consequences.

Be aware of this problem when buying DMSO and do not buy concentrations of less than 99.99% and be sure to use good quality. One way to check is that a pure DMSO solution will turn solid (like ice) below 18ºC. If, when the frozen bottle is turned upside down, little rivulets of water flow through the ice, you probably have bought veterinary grade DMSO; this is only a 90% concentration.

- Women are discouraged from using DMSO during pregnancy or breastfeeding (simply because, should anything go wrong, DMSO would be blamed), even though DMSO is used to preserve frozen human embryos.
- DMSO can interfere with liver function tests and give a false reading. That problem is easily solved by waiting a week after DMSO usage before taking the test
- DMSO is exhaled as DMS and this may give false positives with a ketone breath meter. Some find that the odour is unbearable (I have to say I have not noticed this), in which case use Dr Moran's deodourised preparation (see Useful resources, page 303), which is a bit more expensive.

To find out more about this multi-tasking favourite, I recommend a useful summary by my favourite cardiologist, Dr Gabriella Segura,[11] and the book by Amandha Vollmer, *Healing with DMSO.*[12]

Summary

- DMSO is a safe product when used as described in this chapter, with particular reference to 'Troubleshooting' above...
- DMSO has many desirable properties including:
  - It is anti-inflammatory.
  - It is useful for any autoimmune condition.
  - It is an anticoagulant.
  - It is a painkiller.
  - It improves blood supply.
  - It gets rid of toxic metals.
  - It slows degeneration.
  - It protects mitochondria.

    - It helps to prevent cancer.
    - It protects against radiation.
    - It is antiviral, antibacterial and antifungal.
    - It accelerates healing and repair, so use it for any acute injury, painful area, acute arthritis.
    - It softens connective tissue and scar tissue.
    - It dissolves biofilm.
    - It dissolves kidney stones and gallstones.
- DMSO can be very easily obtained but must be absolutely pure (99.9%%, not 90% veterinary grade).
- It can be taken either orally or via the skin.
- It can be combined with other ingredients such as vitamins and minerals via transdermal preparations.
- Some people experience side effects, but these are abolished, or at least much mitigated, by having Groundhog Chronic (page 232) in place.
- DMSO can skew liver function tests and may affect breath ketone measures.

Chapter 17

Methylene blue for all chronic infections

Methylene blue (MB)* has some properties that make it very desirable for the human body. It is remarkably safe and has been used in humans for decades. This makes it very undesirable for Big Pharma, so its properties are not reported to the medical profession.

There are two major drivers of disease – namely, poor energy delivery mechanisms and chronic inflammation. MB impacts on both. A further problem arises because, as we become ill, the immune system starts to fail, and we acquire not just one but multiple infections. MB has activity against many infections (viral, bacterial and fungal), but what is so interesting is that its effects are activated by far infrared light. This is called photodynamic therapy.

The French national library (Bibliothèque Nationale de France) lists over 100 references on MB, some dating back to 1891.[1]

***Historical note:** Methylene blue is often referred to as 'the first fully synthetic drug used in medicine'. It was first prepared in 1876 by German chemist Heinrich Caro (1834 – 1910). During and after 1891, its use in the treatment of malaria was pioneered by Paul Guttmann (German pathologist, 1834 – 1893) and Paul Ehrlich (Nobel Prize-winning German physician and scientist, 1854 – 1915). It was also used (as an antimalarial) in World War II, where soldiers observed: 'Even at the loo, we see, we pee, navy blue.' Later, clinicians could monitor whether depressed patients were complying with their treatment regimens by observing whether these patients had blue-stained urine.

Table 17.1: Desirable properties of methylene blue (MB)

Action	Disease	Sources and references
Improves mitochondrial function and so energy delivery mechanisms. Can also trap leaking electrons produced by mitochondrial inhibitors and preserve the metabolic rate by bypassing blocked points of electron flow, thus improving mitochondrial respiration	Any disease process associated with poor energy delivery. Chronic fatigue, heart disease, dementia, possibly cancer	Tucker and colleagues (2018) concluded that methylene blue promotes mitochondrial activity and mitigates oxidative stress. In addition, they found that low-dose MB acts as an antioxidant in mitochondria. Furthermore, MB forms water upon exposure to oxygen and this reduces the number of free radicals produced in oxidative phosphorylation.[2]
	Potential for use in stroke, global cerebral ischaemia, Alzheimer's disease, Parkinson's disease, and traumatic brain injury	Tucker and colleagues (2018) also concluded that MB reduced neurodegeneration in conditions such as stroke, global cerebral ischemia, Alzheimer's Disease, Parkinson's Disease and traumatic brain injury.[2]
		In relation to Alzheimer's disease, Ginimuge & Jyothi (2010) concluded that: 'It has been shown to attenuate the formation of amyloid plaques and neurofibrillary tangles and partial repair of impairments in mitochondrial function and cellular metabolism.'[3]
	Chronic fatigue syndrome – due to its effect on mitochondria and possibly through reducing cytokines	Scigliano & Scigliano (2021) concluded that MB is the only compound known to inhibit the excessive production of reactive species and cytokines in Covid-19.[4]

Action	Disease	Sources and references
1880s Nobel laureate Paul Ehrlich discovered methylene Blue as a malaria treatment, and it is considered safe and effective. Current studies have been investigating whether MB treatment alongside other antiparasitic drugs could prevent the parasites from developing drug resistance. Photodynamic therapy using the light-activated antimicrobial agent, MB kills methicillin-resistant *Staphylococcus aureus* (MRSA) in superficial and deep excisional wounds	Any chronic infection may be susceptible to MB. It is biologically plausible that combining MB with far infrared light (ideally at a wavelength of 670 nm which activates MB) may potentiate the antimicrobial action of each other	Ginimuge & Jyothi (2010) concluded: 'Photodynamic therapy using the light activated anti-microbial agent, Methylene blue kills methicillin resistant staphylococcus aureus (MRSA) in superficial and deep excisional wounds. Methylene blue in combination with light also inactivates viral nucleic acid of hepatitis-C and human immunodeficiency virus (HIV-1) and treats cases of resistant plaque psoriasis.'[3] Lu and colleagues (2018) concluded: 'MB was consistently shown to be highly effective in all endemic areas and demonstrated a strong effect on P. falciparum gametocyte reduction.'[5]
MB in combination with light (photodynamic therapy) also inactivates viral nucleic acid of hepatitis C and human immunodeficiency virus (HIV-1), Zika, Ebola, West Nile, Middle East respiratory syndrome, and treats cases of resistant plaque psoriasis	Antiviral	Cagno et al (2021) concluded: 'Our work supports the interest of testing methylene blue in clinical studies to confirm a preventive and/or therapeutic efficacy against both influenza virus H1N1 and SARS-CoV-2 infections.'[6] See also Ginimuge & Jyothi (2010)[3]
Evidence suggests MB is effective against all the herpes viruses including herpes 1 and 2, EBV, CMV and VCZ. Effective against covid 19 (hydroxychloroquine, of proven benefit, is derived from methylene blue)		See the US patent application for more details[7]

Table 17.1 *Cont'd*

Action	Disease	Sources and references
And covid 19		Hamidi-Alamdari and colleagues (2021) concluded that adding MB to already existing treatment protocols improved oxygen saturation levels in Covid-19 patients and reduced respiratory distress and that this lead to shorter hospital stays and lower mortality rates.[8] Neha Dabholkar and colleagues described MB as a 'magic bullet' for Covid-19 treatment[9]
An antifungal agent and may inhibit candida by causing mitochondrial dysfunction in this species	Antifungal	See the paper by Ansair and colleagues (2016)[11]
Binds to methaemoglobin and converts it to a more efficient form, thereby improving the symptoms of methemoglobinaemia	Carbon monoxide poisoning	See the article and links on SelfDecode[10]
A monoamine oxidase inhibitor	Depression: the dose used is very small – just 15 mg per day	Naylor and colleagues (1987) concluded that MB, at a dose of 15 mg daily, and used over a three-week period, gave improvements over and above placebo in severe depressive illness[12]

How to tackle any chronic infection

So, to tackle any chronic infection, this is the programme:

- Start with Groundhog Chronic (PK diet, sort out the fermenting gut, supplements, detox, sort out the thyroid and adrenal glands – Appendix 1).
- Then DMSO (Chapter 16).
- Then MB.

- Then far infrared (FIR) light (Chapter 18). Both DMSO and MB are activated by FIR light.

This is a package which is biologically plausible, intrinsically safe and very affordable. Build up very slowly to mitigate detox and die-off (DDD) reactions (Appendix 2).

Dose of MB

MB should always be taken in low doses. The safe low dose is 1-2 mg per kg of body weight.

Regardless of body weight, start with 10 mg per day.

Indeed, it is so safe it can be used directly into a vein, in doses of 15 mg per kg of body weight.

Always purchase pharmaceutical grade MB (this is clean and free from impurities). You could start by purchasing a 1% solution but since most products come in small volumes you will get through this very quickly. As your need for MB increases, it is much more economical to purchase it as the pure powder (see Useful resources, page 303). Make sure this is British Pharmaceutical standard (it will have BP 73 on it so it conforms to the standards set in 1973). It may also be marked 'Harmful if swallowed'. That simply reflects the fact that the powder is pure and needs to be diluted with water.

This comes in a 10-gram pot (approximate cost from my website, £11 at the time of going to press). Take the whole pot and dissolve the contents in 1000 ml (1 litre) of water. This gives a 1% solution – that is, 10 mg/ml. So, for a daily dose of 120 mg (2 mg per kg body weight) or 12 ml this would last 80 days. (This makes it a perfect treatment for my PBs – see page xvi!) Be careful mixing it up. Should you spill the blue crystals or liquid (and I have) you will spend the rest of your day washing out the colour. I did! Start with 1 ml per day in a single dose at night. Put this into a large glass of water. I suggest you also add 1-2 g ascorbic acid; this converts much of the MB to leucoMB which is colourless. This may take several minutes but you get round the tooth/tongue staining issue. Drink the pale blue solution. In the body MB alternates between MB and leucoMB as it donates or accepts electrons. This explains the many desirable actions of MB. Expect to pee blue. (To avoid the blue staining your teeth, you can also drink the solution through a straw.)

Increase the dose in 10 mg steps – that is, 1 ml increments depending on how you tolerated this.

A 60-kg person could end up on 6 ml per day for 1 mg per kg, or 12 ml per day for 2 mg/kg.

For how long to use MB, see Chapter 22 (page 213).

Caution with MB

MB is a monoamine oxidase inhibitor (MAOI) which partly explains its antidepressive and antianxiety effects.[13]

MAOIs can cause dangerous interactions with certain foods and beverages so when you're taking MB you'll need to avoid foods containing high levels of tyramine — an amino acid that regulates blood pressure. These include aged cheeses, sauerkraut, cured meats, draft beer and fermented soy products (for example, soy sauce, miso and tofu). The interaction of tyramine with MAOIs can cause dangerously high blood pressure. Also take care with coffee, chocolate and broad beans among other foods.[14]

Alcoholic drinks must be tyramine free so avoid beer, wine, port and sherry. Spirits (gin, rum, vodka, whisky) and cider are safe in modest amounts.

MAOIs can also cause serious reactions when you take them with certain medications, such as other antidepressants, certain pain drugs, certain cold and allergy medications, amphetamines, blood pressure drugs, migraine drugs, some antibiotics or antifungals, recreational drugs, tegretol, disulphiram and some herbal supplements, such as St John's wort and ginseng.

If you are taking *any* medication, do check for interactions with MAOIs.[15]

Conclusion

For more, useful information about MB, take a look at the recent release from the Orthomolecular Medicine News Service (OMNS)[16] Their link for a free subscription is:

http://orthomolecular.org/subscribe.html

and their archive link is:

http://orthomolecular.org/resources/omns/index.shtml

Summary

- Methylene blue has many desirable properties including:
  - It improves mitochondrial function and so energy delivery mechanisms.
  - It treats malaria and has antiparasitic, antibacterial, antifungal and antiviral properties, including against Covid-19.
  - It has antidepressant effects.
- Methylene blue can be easily obtained and used.
- There are some advisory notes – e.g. care with certain food types because it is a monoamine oxidase inhibitor.

Chapter 18

Photodynamic* therapy

We know that light and heat kill many infections (see our book *The Infection Game*). We also know that if you have one infection then it is very likely there are other infections and therefore the logical starting point is a broad-spectrum antimicrobial to reduce the load of all. What is so interesting is that methylene blue (MB) is activated by light (see Chapter 17). Since both MB and light are inexpensive, very safe and available to all, I can see this combination becoming another of my favourite multi-tasking tools. Light has many other wonderful properties. These include:

- **Improved mitochondrial function** which, in turn, improves energy delivery mechanisms so that the immune system has the energy to fight infection.
- **Improved antioxidant status** to reduce the 'friendly fire' free radical damage which is an inevitable result of the immune system killing microbes.
- **Penetrates deeply into the tissue** at least several centimetres. This means that all body tissues can be accessed. Of course, any infection that is carried in the bloodstream will be easily accessed by light as some blood returns to the heart via superficial veins.

There are many studies showing that light is efficacious. It multi-tasks and is effective for treating many other conditions that are associated with infectious disease (in combination

*__Linguistic note:__ The commonly used English language prefix, 'photo' is derived from the Greek, *phos* ('light') whose genitive (i.e. possessive) form is 'photos' (meaning 'of light'). 'Dynamic' also derives from a Greek word, *dynamis*, meaning force or power. So, 'photodynamic' translates in Greek as 'the power of light', and as we shall see, this is, indeed, a very apt description.

with Groundhog Chronic – Appendix 1). Thank you, Dr James Laporta, for opening my eyes to these possibilities.

Table 18.1: The benefits of light

Which	Why and how	Sources and references
Parkinson's disease (PD) and dementia Traumatic brain injury Autism	Prevents neurodegeneration. Most studies use near infrared light	Johnstone and colleagues (2015) concluded: 'Red to infrared light therapy (λ = 600-1070 nm), and in particular light in the near infrared (NIr) range, is emerging as a safe and effective therapy that is capable of arresting neuronal death. Previous studies have used NIr to treat tissue stressed by hypoxia, toxic insult, genetic mutation and mitochondrial dysfunction with much success. Here we propose NIr therapy as a neuroprotective or disease-modifying treatment for Alzheimer's and Parkinson's patients'[1]
	Improves mitochondrial function and dopaminergic cell longevity Activates stem cells Harmonises brain waves Improves circulation	The study by Johnstone and colleagues (2015) references a further 122 studies supporting the stated benefits.[1] I have chosen five of these studies as representative of these benefits[2, 3, 4, 5, 6]
	Dementia and PD are infection driven	See Chapter 15 (page 146) and our book *The Infection Game* AND microbes from the abnormal microbiome
	Photodynamic therapy (PDT) works in practice when a transcranial laser helmet is used with light at 810 nm wavelength	Ann Liebert and colleagues (2021) concluded: 'PBM was shown to be a safe and potentially effective treatment for a range of clinical signs and symptoms of PD. Improvements were maintained for as long as treatment continued, for up to one year in a neurodegenerative disease where decline is typically expected. Home treatment of PD by the person themselves or with the help of a carer might be an effective therapy option. The results of this study indicate that a large RCT is warranted'[7]

Table 18.1 *Cont'd*

Which	Why and how	Sources and references
	Use with curcumin	Curcumin is additionally helpful. RB Mythri and MM Srinivas (2012) concluded that curcumin exhibits antioxidant, anti-inflammatory and anticancer action, and given that it crosses the blood-brain barrier, it additionally shows neuroprotective action in neurological disease. In particular, the authors concluded strong efficacy, as demonstrated in many studies, for Parkinson's disease (PD).[8]
	Use with high-dose thiamine e.g. benfotiamine 300 mg daily – this is fat-soluble so easily crosses the blood-brain barrier; take it with a fatty meal	Thiamine is additionally helpful. Antonio Costantini and colleagues (2013) concluded that it led to improvements in the Unified Parkinson's Disease Rating Scale ranging from around 30% to as high as 77%. The authors then stated that it was reasonable to infer that severe thiamine deficiency was causing neuronal damage in centres that are typically affected in PD.[9]
Parkinson's disease	More evidence for thiamine	Antonio Costantini and colleagues (2015) concluded that, once again, thiamine treatment led to improvements in the Unified Parkinson's Disease Rating Scale of around 40% on average and that these improvements occurred within three months of starting treatment and that such improvements remained stable over time. Indeed, some patients, with a milder phenotype, had complete clinical recovery.[10]
Dementia		Farzad Salehpour and colleagues (2021) concluded that, after reviewing 36 studies, all reported positive results, with a lack of adverse side effects.[11]

Which	Why and how	Sources and references
Traumatic brain injury		Maria Gabriela Figueiro Longo and colleagues (2020) concluded: 'In this randomized clinical trial, low level laser therapy (LLLT) was feasible in all patients and did not exhibit any adverse events. Light therapy altered multiple diffusion tensor parameters in a statistically significant manner in the late subacute stage. This study provides the first human evidence to date that light therapy engages neural substrates that play a role in the pathophysiologic factors of moderate TBI.'[12]
Autism		Gerry Leisman and colleagues (2018) concluded that low laser therapy could be an effective treatment tool for autistic spectrum disorder in children and adolescents. They noted that positive behavioural changes were seen and that these were maintained, and in some case, improved over time.[13]
Bacterial infection		Qinyu Han and colleagues (2021) concluded that near infrared light irradiation acts as an effective disinfectant for bacteria and is a candidate for further investigation for eradicating multidrug resistant bacteria and inhibiting antibiotic resistance in general.[14]
Inflam-mation	Both near and far infrared are helpful. Both impact the fourth phase of water	Chih-Ching Lin and colleagues (2008) concluded that far infrared therapy has a strong anti-inflammatory effect and that this may play a crucial role in preserving blood flow in arteriovenous fistula in haemodialysis patients.[15]
Any condition associated with sticky blood	PDT supplies the energy for water molecules to 'honeycomb' as gel water – this charges all membranes negatively so blood cells repel each other and do not stick	See *The Fourth Phase of Water* by Gerald Pollack.[16]
Cancer	PDT is directly toxic to cancer cells	See Cancer Research UK.[17]

Table 18.1 *Cont'd*

Which	Why and how	Sources and references
	PDT can be used with a light-sensitive drugs such as methylene blue (see Chapter 17)	Ancély F Dos Santos and colleagues (2017) concluded: 'Finally, our observations underscore the potential of MB-PDT as a highly efficient strategy which could use as a powerful adjunct therapy to surgery of breast tumours, and possibly other types of tumours, to safely increase the eradication rate of microscopic residual disease and thus minimizing the chance of both local and metastatic recurrence.'[18]

How to put this all in place

- First establish Groundhog Chronic (see Appendix 1). There is no point killing infections if you are feeding the little wretches with sugar and carbs, and there is no point using anti-inflammatory interventions if you are driving inflammation with sugar and carbs. This is an arms race – it is not a battle, it is a war!
- Start with DMSO (see Chapter 16).
- Then add in methylene blue (see Chapter 17).
- Then add in light.

Which device?

The best source of light is sunshine, but this is not readily available if you live in the UK, and not convenient if you work at a desk. Sunbathe all you can without burning whenever you get the chance – do not use sunscreens – and/or find a device that is convenient and delivers the correct wavelength of light to the right area of the body for a reasonable length of time. Yes, we are all on a steep learning curve (in fact I have never been off such). The joy is that near infrared (NIF) and far infrared (FIR) radiation are so safe that we do not have to be too precise – we can play it by ear.

Start low, go slow and expect die-off and detox (DDD) reactions (see Appendix 2). Dr James Laporta developed a hat for transcranial use that uses NIF light at 810 nm, which he describes as an 'LED helmet'. NIR light is a wavelength just beyond visible at 780 nm to 1000 nm; it does not warm and penetrates deep into muscles, organs and bones. FIR is a wavelength of 3000 nm to 1,000,000 nm and penetrates even deeper and is warming.

There is a wide range of devices, many costing less that £100 at the time of going to press, that deliver NIR light. My personal choice would be for a belt (see Useful resources, page 303) so that I could wear it but still move around to get jobs done. Choose one that suits your lifestyle.

[†]**Aside by Craig:** Is there a power greater than the Power of Light? Perhaps the Power of Love? And this reminds me of that classic film moment in *Back to the Future* when to the theme tune, 'The Power of Love' (by Huey Lewis and the News), Jennifer Parker (Claudia Wells) hands her phone number written on a 'Save the Clock Tower' flyer to Marty McFly (Michael J Fox) and just above her number, she has written 'I love You'. The look on Marty's face says it all! And as an aside to this aside, Jennifer's phone number is 555-4823. The prefix 555 is used in many (American) films and, indeed, this was encouraged by US telephone companies – these numbers either did not exist or were used for directory services and so, by using these numbers, the film makers did not risk giving out private numbers. Nowadays, only 555-0100 through to 555-0199 are specifically reserved for fictional use; the other numbers have been reserved for actual assignment. Further examples of the use of 555 prefixes are that Jim Rockford's phone number in the American detective television series *The Rockford Files* was (311) 555-2368, as was one of Jaime Sommers' private numbers in *The Bionic Woman*; and as a seven-digit call, 555-2368 reached *The Ghostbusters*! There are many, many more… across other countries as well. The interested reader should see https://en.wikipedia.org/wiki/Fictitious_telephone_number

Summary

- Photodynamic therapy (PDT)
    - improves mitochondrial function
    - which, in turn, improves energy delivery mechanisms so that the immune system has the energy to fight infection
    - improves antioxidant status
    - is anti-inflammatory
    - penetrates deeply into the tissues
    - is directly toxic to many microbes.
- PDT has been shown to be effective for:
    - Parkinson's disease (PD) and dementia
    - Traumatic brain injury
    - Autism
    - Bacterial infection
    - Cancer
    - Inflammation – and 'sticky blood'.
- Use PDT with DMSO and methylene blue for best effect, putting Groundhog Chronic (page 240) in place before all else, as always.
- Many devices can deliver the required light – belts for example are very convenient (see Useful resources, page 303).

Chapter 19

Reprogramming the immune system with micro-immunotherapy (MIT)

Micro-immunotherapy (MIT)* is fast proving to be a useful tool. It is to the immune system what psychotherapy is to the brain – it retrains it to behave appropriately. I think that just as the brain has states and moods, so does the immune system. The happy brain has a happy immune system (by which I mean it is relaxed and does not react to every incitant); the anxious brain has an anxious immune system (it fires off at random all over the place with allergy and autoimmunity) and the depressed brain has a depressed immune system ('can't be bothered' to fight, so allows infections to run amok). This helps to explain which micro-immunotherapy remedies to use.

***Linguistic note:** Micro-immunotherapy is an example of a compound and/or portmanteau word. Compound words are words that join full words together and portmanteau words are words that join together full words or parts of words. The Germans are very good at it.

- *Geschwindigkeitsbeschränkungen*, meaning speed limits.
- *Handschuhschneeballwerfer* meaning a person who wears gloves to throw snowballs.
- *Donaudampfschiffahrtselektrizitätenhauptbetriebswerkbauunterbeamtengesellschaft* - the association for subordinate officials of the head office management of the Danube steamboat electrical services.
- *Sitzpinkler* – a man who pees sitting down. Isn't that a *great* word?

There are some interesting facts about where in the world men pee sitting down and where it is more usual to stand – in the UK, standing is more usual; in Germany, men most often sit so they are *Sitzpinklers*! (I know – I have pluralised that incorrectly.) See this map of Europe: https://mapsontheweb.zoom-maps.com/post/654959702557507584/sit-or-stand-in-which-countries-in-europe-men.

MIT can also reduce the infectious load

Viruses replicate by hijacking the protein synthesising mechanisms within cells. They achieve this by inserting themselves into the cells' DNA so that it creates viruses. Jolly clever! MIT competes with viral proteins for these sites and so the cell makes false virus which is inactive. Instead of making a scorpion with a sting in the tail, the cell makes a scorpion with a fluffy tail. It's useless.

MIT acts on the brain by the same mechanisms with which it acts on the immune system. We want remedies that are appropriate to the clinical picture.

How to use MIT

1. Use MIT to regulate energy delivery mechanisms

Mitochondria are intelligent and there is much communication with the immune system. We know mitochondria are responsible for cell suicide (apoptosis) and are central players in autoimmunity. There is a logical progression to using MIT, which can be employed in addition to Groundhog Chronic (see page 240).

Table 19.1: Which remedies are appropriate to the clinical picture

Clinical picture	Remedy
With severe physical fatigue, especially when the patient does not tolerate interventions and/or gets nasty die-off and detox (DDD) reactions. When mitochondria are not responding to the mitochondrial package of treatment; they seem to have gone into 'hibernation'. This may be part of what Robert Naviaux called the 'cell danger response': 'the evolutionarily conserved metabolic response that protects hosts from harm. It is triggered by encounters with chemical, physical, or biological threats that exceed the cellular capacity for homeostasis.'[1] Additionally useful where there is autoimmunity	MIREG
With mental stress and anxiety (I suspect these are symptoms the brain gives us when it knows it does not have the energy to deal with demands)	MISEN

Marked foggy brain – patients feel they are going demented. (I suspect these are symptoms of inflammation in the brain)	DEP MEM-SENIOR
The inflamed brain that does not sleep	SLEEP REG

2. Use MIT to regulate the immune system

If the immune system is in an overactive state (anxious and inflamed) then there is 'friendly fire'. In this event, use remedies that focus that activity.

On the other hand, if the immune system is fatigued ('can't be bothered' or does not have the energy to fight) then you do not want remedies that squash it. You need remedies that stimulate.

So, the first question to ask is if the immune system is overactive (anxious or inflamed) or underactive (depressed).

Table 19.2: The signs and symptoms of an overactive and underactive immune system

Overactive (anxious and inflamed)	**Underactive (depressed and fatigued)**	**For further info:**
20% are overactive	80% are underactive	
Symptoms of inflammation	None, or few symptoms	Chapter 10
High white cell count	Low white cell count	Appendix 3
High markers of inflammation (ESR, CRP, plasma viscosity)	Low markers of inflammation	Appendix 3
High ferritin	Normal or low ferritin	Appendix 3

If you are not sure whether you are inflamed or not, then go for underactive – 80% are.

There are clinical tests that can be done as a guide. For these, you need an experienced practitioner available through Natural Health Worldwide (see Useful resources, page 303).

Alternatively, if you find that you are made worse by a remedy, then try one that does the opposite.

Underactive immune system

If the clinical picture is underactive (80% of cases), fatigued, depressed and 'cannot be bothered' to fight AND/OR to reduce the infectious load follow the guidance in Table 19.3. This makes the remedies in Table 19.3 good for an acute infection also.

Some patients need more than one remedy. In this event, remedies should be separated by at least 30 minutes.

Table 19.3: Remedies for the underactive immune system

Infective organism	Notes	Remedy
ME following Covid infection or Covid vaccinations i.e. long Covid (LC) OR not sure what the infection is	For acute infection this can be used up to four times daily Also good for those who seem to pick up every microbe going around.	EID
Epstein Barr virus (aka glandular fever or mononucleosis). EBV is a really nasty virus, a common trigger of ME, multiple sclerosis, autoimmunity and many cancers	In LC there is often reactivation of underlying viruses, especially EBV. Chen and colleagues (2019) found: 'EBV seropositivity was associated with fever and increased inflammation.'[2] Jeffrey Gold and colleagues (2021) concluded that many long Covid symptoms may be related to EBV reactivation as a result of inflammation initially caused by acute Covid-19 infection, rather than as a result of the ongoing effects of Covid-19 infection itself.[3] Common things are common! So, this is a widely used remedy	EBV

Infective organism	Notes	Remedy
Cytomegalovirus	Ditto above, and Michael J Peluso and colleagues (2022) concluded that: 'participants who had serologic evidence of prior CMV infection were less likely to develop neurocognitive LC (OR† 0.52) and tended to have less severe (>5 symptoms reported) LC (OR 0.44)' [than those with chronic EBV] *but* it was still a risk factor[4]	CMV
Herpes I or II	This is the first remedy that gynaecologists on the Continent use for acute and chronic herpes. It is of proven benefit	HERP
Chicken pox or shingles	This is often associated with pain syndromes	ZONA
Chlamydia or mycoplasma		CHLA
Hepatitis B or C		HC
Papilloma virus (HPV)	This is the first remedy that gynaecologists on the Continent use. It is of proven benefit	PAPI
Lyme disease	There is no specific remedy, but Lyme often drives autoimmunity	See below

Overactive immune system

If the clinical picture suggests that the immune system is overactive and anxious (20% of patients) then follow the recommendations in Table 19.4. Friendly fire will be causing widespread, useless and destructive damage. We want focus.

†**Statistical note:** OR = Odds Ratio – the strength of association between, for example, severe LC and CMV (cytomegalovirus) was 0.44 – the higher the OR, the stronger the association. CMV is often associated with gut symptoms.

Table 19.4: Remedies for the overactive immune system

Type of overactivity	Notes	Suggested remedy
Overactive immune system with pain (especially acute symptoms)	With acute symptoms use this up to four times daily, in strict numerical order	ARTH
Overactive immune system with autoimmunity (especially chronic symptoms)	There are over 100 autoimmune disorders, so the majority are not tested for. Spike protein resembles at least 80 human proteins so there is potential to switch on autoimmunity	INFLAM
Overactive immune system with allergy	Does not switch off allergy so much as render the whole system generally less reactive	ALLERG
Inflammatory bowel disease (Crohn's and ulcerative colitis)		MICI
Overactive immune system *plus* ME	If you are not sure if you are overactive or underactive, then this is a safe start – at least you will not risk making yourself/the person worse	XFS

How to take MIT

ALWAYS take capsules in strict numerical-order, 10-capsule cycles. Each 10-capsule cycle represents a course.

For acute infections one can take the course at an accelerated rate of up to 4 capsules daily. Again, they must be taken in strict order. Therefore 10 capsules will last 2.5 days. Again, they must be taken as below, under the tongue, 30 minutes away from food or water.

Take on rising by pouring the contents of 1 capsule under the tongue and letting it dissolve. Do not eat or drink for at least 30 minutes. Do not swallow the capsule contents

– hold under the tongue until they dissolve away. It contains some lactose and sucrose as an excipient, but the amounts are tiny and rarely cause problems.

You can take more than one course of MIT, but capsules must be separated by 30 minutes as above.

Once MIT is working well, it is suggested that low-dose maintenance be used for the long term at the rate of 10 capsules for the first 10 days of each month (leaving a break of three weeks between each cycle of treatment).

For chronic disease you must commit to at least 3 months of therapy.

How to access MIT

To access MIT, go through Natural Health Worldwide (see Useful resources, page 303).

FIRST put in place Groundhog Chronic and give this time to take effect.

THEN, if the clinical picture fits as described above, the practitioner can supply (or get in touch with me to source).

More information

Please see Micro-Immunotherapy International Medical Experience at www.micro-immunotherapy.com
This website includes a list of 31 medical and scientific papers concerning MIT.[5]

Summary

- MIT can help if Ground Chronic is fully in place and things are still not improving or not improving quickly enough.
- MIT can help with:
  - energy delivery mechanisms.
  - regulating the immune system.
  - reducing the infectious load.
  - specific remedies for particular diseases.

Chapter 20

Reducing the infectious load

Specific antivirals, antimicrobials and antifungals

Of course, we all want to be told that we have a single infection which will need an antimicrobial and then all will be well. That is rarely the case. So often I see patients who have spent a small fortune on antibiotics for Lyme, antifungals for yeast or antivirals for chronic EBV but are no better. It is not that they have been mistreated; it is simply that all these antimicrobials reduce the infectious load, and it is up to the immune system to do the rest. If the immune system does not have the energy, the raw materials or the direction to act, then the infections will simply bounce back once the course of antimicrobials has been completed. Furthermore, co-infections will not have been addressed.

Restoring health is not a battle. It is a war – a war that we know we shall eventually lose, but I will settle for losing aged 100. I hope then to sail off to another world on addiction – at medical school the most prescribed was 'Brompton Cocktail'* – a mixture of gin, morphine and cocaine.

So, if despite all that has gone before, or perhaps during, you would like to do some tests to see if you are harbouring a chronic infection this chapter gives a summary. Diagnosis is the starting point to treatment, but I cannot cover the whole of infectious disease in

*__Medical note:__ The Brompton cocktail was named after the Royal Brompton Hospital in London, England, where the formulation of this mixture was standardised in the late 1920s for patients, primarily with cancer. Its use is rare these days, but it was used frequently in the late 19th and early 20th Centuries.

one chapter – you need to read our book *The Infection Game* for details of regimes and specific antimicrobials.

Principles of diagnosis of chronic 'stealth' infections – which tests?

There may be clues from the clinical picture (see Table 20.1), but a definite diagnosis will require laboratory tests. These are expensive, but we can increase the chances of a positive diagnosis by first considering symptoms and signs.

A vital and powerful symptom of a chronic stealth infection is failure to respond to Groundhog interventions. Regardless of whether you do or do not test positive for a chronic stealth infection, Groundhog must be in place for long-term good health, especially with old crones like me – so just do it, do it well and do it now. Indeed, I know that many of my patients must have been cured through Groundhog interventions alone. I say that because these stealth infections are common, so many of my patients who have recovered are likely, unknowingly, to have suffered from them.

Symptoms and signs of, and tests for, chronic infection

Start with the time when the symptoms began, which may be decades before. The list in Table 20.1 is not comprehensive but is put in order of probability based on my clinical experience. From there, move on to tests.

- For the best chance of making the diagnosis, you need tests of the humoral response (antibody tests) and the cellular response (Elispot tests).
- Raised IgM levels point to an acute infection.
- Raised IgG levels point to a past infection BUT if the antibody titre is five times higher than the reference range that may indicate a chronic infection.
- Raised IgA levels point to a mucosal surface infection, such as mycoplasma.
- Tests are available through labs at www.naturalhealthworldwide.com (see Useful resources, page 303).

Table 20.1: When and which tests are worth doing for chronic infection

How symptoms started	Possible diagnosis	Useful tests to support diagnosis in order of priority
With Covid-19 or the mRNA vaccine	Long Covid	SARS Covid 2 ELISA Armin labs (known as AONM (Academy of Nutritional Medicine) in the UK)
Sudden 'flu-like illness, fever, malaise. Feeling ghastly and unable to do anything let alone work. Bedbound for some days. Perhaps swollen glands in neck, armpits, groin. Perhaps went a bit yellow. Perhaps pericarditis and chest pain. At the time blood tests may have been 'A bit wrong but nothing to worry about'	HHV4 (glandular fever) known as 'infectious mononucleosis', or just 'mono' in the US	Armin laboratory tests: Elispot, IgG antibody titre, IgM antibody titre, DNA by PCR. A raised IgG is typically interpreted as evidence of past exposure ergo no treatment necessary, but it does not exclude the possibility that a microbe is driving pathology
Ditto	HHV6 roseola	IgG/IgM antibodies DNA PCR
Ditto	Coxsackie virus	IgG/IgA antibodies
Ditto	HHV5 Cytomegalovirus (CMV)	Elispot (Armin)
Above with localising signs e.g. shingles, chickenpox Pain syndromes Cold sores and genital herpes are also herpes virus but rarely trigger CFS/ME	Other herpes viruses. All herpes viruses target the brain and immune system. Once in the body all herpes viruses persist for life	Elispot for varicella zoster (shingles chicken pox). Elispot HSV1 HSV2. IgG antibody titre
Vaccination – I estimate that one in 10 of my CFS/ME patients have their disease triggered or worsened by vaccination. Covid mRNA gene therapy 'vaccines' are especially pernicious		

Table 20.1 *Cont'd*

How symptoms started	**Possible diagnosis**	**Useful tests to support diagnosis in order of priority**
	These are designed to switch on the immune system with the potential to trigger autoimmunity and allergy	There may be positive IgG titres to virus
	We know some retroviruses have been present in vaccination such as SV 40. The jury is still out with respect to XMRV	Impossible to get retroviral tests done (except HIV)
Acute gastroenteritis (or indeed any gut symptom such as pain, bloating, reflux, diarrhoea, constipation, abnormally formed stools)	Fermenting gut. Inflammatory bowel disease (*Mycobacterium avium paratuberculosis* – potential trigger for Crohn's disease). Parasite or unfriendly gut microbes e.g. *H pylori*, giardia, *Amoebiasis blastocystis hominis*	Comprehensive digestive stool analysis e.g. available from Doctors Data or Genova or from Smart Nutrition, without the need for practitioner referral (see page 303). I know of no commercial test for MAP
Possibly a tick bite and bull's eye rash but probably none such. As with borrelia, babesia and bartonella, any insect bite could transmit many infections. Possibly rash and arthritic condition. Often no clear onset	Lyme disease (*Borrelia burgdorferi*) *Borrelia myamotoi*	Armin labs: Elispot Seraspot (Often antibody tests are negative – this does not exclude the diagnosis)
As with borrelia, could be acquired through insect bites. Virtually all mammals harbour bartonella. Classically follows cat scratch ('cat scratch fever'), but absence of such does not exclude the diagnosis	Bartonella – may cause a PUO – pyrexia of unknown origin, sometimes referred to as fever of unknown origin (FUO)	Armin: Elispot IgG/IgM antibodies DNA PCR
Insect bites	Babesia – may cause a PUO	Armin: Elispot IgG/IgM antibodies. Babesia DNA PCR

How symptoms started	Possible diagnosis	Useful tests to support diagnosis in order of priority
	Rickettsia	Elispot: Ehrlichia Elispot: Anaplasma
	Yersinia	Elispot: Yersinia
Chest infection or pneumonia (may be atypical 'walking pneumonia' i.e. the patient is not very ill). I seem to be seeing many new cases	*Mycoplasma pneumoniae*	IgG antibodies
Ditto	*Chlamydia pneumoniae*	Elispot: IgG antibodies
Sexually transmitted disease	Chlamydia trachomatis HIV, hepatitis C, syphilis, herpes, HPV, gonorrhoea, trichomonas, bacterial vaginosis	Get screening tests at a Special Clinic Elispot IgG antibodies
Recurrent chest, upper respiratory or sinus infections	Chronic septic focus e.g. bronchiectasis Fungal infection such as aspergillosis	Chest X-ray, sputum sample (but often false negatives). Aspergillus precipitation test. IgG IgM and IgA antibodies
Joint pains and arthritis	Inflammation driven by allergy to microbes from the fermenting gut OR allergy to a virus – so called 'reactive arthritis'	No direct tests. Autoantibody studies may help. Investigations for the fermenting gut: Comprehensive digestive stool analysis e.g. Doctors Data or Genova or from Smart Nutrition, without the need for practitioner referral (see page 303)

Current symptoms and signs

Chronic infections often start with local symptoms of inflammation such as sore throat, head cold, chest infection, gastroenteritis, urinary tract infection or whatever, but as the microbe makes itself comfortably at home in your body then the symptoms become more general and indeed may start to trigger pathology. Many chronic so-called 'degenerative' conditions we know are driven by infection. This includes most cases of dementia (herpes viruses, Lyme), Parkinson's (Lyme), many cases of autoimmunity, cancer, arterial disease, arthritis and of course CFS, ME and LC. Indeed, with any inflammatory pathology always think and look for an infectious cause.

When I was at medical school, I learned that syphilis was the great mimic because it can cause almost any pathology. Syphilis had to be thought of in almost every differential diagnosis. Lyme too is a spirochete (a spiral shaped bacterium) with similar potential for damage and mimicry. In a case report Ahmet Burakgazi demonstrates this possibility for mimicry; he describes how he initially diagnosed amyotrophic lateral sclerosis (ALS – a form of motor neurone disease) but blood serology indicated the possibility of Lyme disease, and subsequent treatment with doxycycline (an antibiotic used in the treatment of Lyme disease) resolved the case completely – the patient recovered and the results of electrodiagnostic tests were clear.[1] In other words, as well as the current signs and symptoms as above, virtually any pathology can be mimicked by Lyme and so one has to be very circumspect.

Interpretation of tests

No test is perfect – all must be interpreted in the light of that patient's history… and all patients are unique. This is what makes medicine an art as much as a science. So much modern Western medicine has been condensed to simple algorithms based on a drug end result so that real pathology is missed. Patients suffer and die needlessly. Nowhere is this a greater issue than the interpretation of tests. Any result is taken as absolute. So often I see patients who are told that all the tests are normal, so they are either not ill or hypochondriacs. Nowhere is this worse than in the field of myalgic encephalitis.

There are several possible mechanisms that form the basis of tests to decide if chronic infection is present:

- A false negative result means: this does not exclude infection.
- A false positive result means: there may be, or has been, microbe exposure but it is no longer a clinical problem.

A mathematical view of what makes a good test

Imagine, says Craig, a test for a microbe where:

- For people that really do have the microbe present, the test says 'Yes' 80% of the time.
- For people that do not have the microbe present, the test says 'Yes' 10% of the time ('false positive').

This may seem like quite a good test, but it really isn't. Take a look at Table 20.2:

Table 20.2: False negatives and positives of this test

State/Test result	**Test says 'Yes'**	**Test says 'No'**
Has microbe	80%	20% (false negative)
Doesn't have microbe	10% (false positive)	90%

There are many ways to work out how good this test is, including the use of Bayes Theorem on Conditional Probability but we don't need that. Instead:

- Imagine 1000 people take this test.
- Imagine 1% of the population actually has this microbe present.
- Imagine you test positive – what are the chances do you think that you have the microbe present? Think NOW of what you think the chances are, roughly, of your having the microbe, if you test positive. Write it down. Gosh, this is like a magic show, or card trick!

Solution:

- Of 1000 people, only 10 really have the microbe (1% of 1000 is 10).
- The test is 80% right for people who have the microbe, so it will get eight of those 10 right.
- But 990 do not have the microbe, and the test will say 'Yes' to 10% of them, which is 99 people it says 'Yes' to wrongly (false positive).
- So out of 1000 people the test says 'Yes' to (8 + 99) = 107 people.

This is shown in Table 20.3.

Table 20.3: Accuracy of this test

State/Test	1% have it	Test says 'Yes'	Test says 'No'
Has microbe	10	8	2
Doesn't have microbe	990	99	891
Totals	1000	107	893

So, 107 people get a 'Yes' but only eight of those really have the microbe:
We have 8/107 = about 7%. So, even though your test said 'Yes', it is only 7% likely that you have the microbe present.

Is this percentage smaller or larger than the figure you guessed earlier? For me, it is much smaller than I guessed. Yes, even mathematicians can be fooled by numbers!

Why is this percentage so low – that is to say, why is it that, even though the test is positive, the chances of having the microbe are so low? It is all about how the various percentages above interplay with each other but, in general terms, if the overall prevalence of the microbe is low (here it is 1% and so, yes, that is low) then you are more likely to have problems like this. But also, the rates of false positives and false negatives play important roles in how much reliance you can put on test results. In other words, it is difficult to know whether you can trust a test result!

So, what do we do? This is, again, where medicine is as much an art as a science. Table 20.4 summarises situations where you can 'believe' test results, and also those where you need to have a good degree of suspicion.

You may need different tests for different microbes depending on where it is living in the body, and whether the immune system is fighting it with antibodies or with white cell foot soldiers.

Table 20.4: Believability of test results

Test	Mechanism	Notes
Can that microbe be seen or grown in tissue culture?	Not all can be – viruses cannot be grown in culture	False negative results are common. A positive result makes it very likely you are harbouring that microbe
PCR (polymerase chain reaction)	If positive, then that microbe *is* present	BUT false negatives abound. You will only get a positive result if the microbe you are looking for is present in the tissue sample that has been taken
	AND if there are too many cycles of PCR, then you can 'find' almost anything!	This was the case with Covid-19 where a cycle threshold of 25 was considered reliable. However, many used cycle thresholds that were higher so rendering the test unreliable
Are there IgM antibodies to that microbe?	This is part of the acute immune response	If positive, then the immune system is fighting that microbe. BUT false negatives abound with 'stealth' infections
Are there IgG antibodies to that microbe?	This forms part of immune memory	We commonly see a positive result which may well mean all is well – i.e. that microbe has been dealt with and kicked into touch by the immune system
		However, sometimes there are very high IgG responses which may suggest the immune system is still fighting a battle†
Are there IgA antibodies to that microbe?	Tests only apply to microbes living on mucous membranes such as *Mycoplasma pneumoniae*	False negatives possible

Table 20.4 *Cont'd*

Test	Mechanism	Notes
Elispot testing looks at how the white T cell soldiers are reacting with cytokines to a particular microbe. Also known as 'lymphocyte transformation test' because the normally quiet white cell soldiers transform into fighting lunatics!	This test is very sensitive, specific and clinically relevant	A positive result means the immune system is fighting that infection. This is a very good test for infection with: • a high level of sensitivity (i.e. false negatives are uncommon) and • a high level of specificity (i.e. it is the microbe you are looking at and not another)
White cell counts	May be high during acute infection	Help these with Groundhog Acute
	May be low with chronic infection...	...as the immune system becomes exhausted because it is running out of raw materials or energy. Treat this with Groundhog Chronic (see page 240)

A general rule of thumb amongst clinicians is that, if the antibody titre is five times higher than baseline, then consider an antiviral strategy. What is so interesting is that Dr Lerner showed that the antiviral titre (EBV nuclear antigen and EBV viral capsid antigen) fell with effective treatment and that this was paralleled by clinical

[†]**Note about testing:** For example, finding a high IgG antibody titre is generally thought to be simply evidence of past infection. However, we know that all herpes viruses persist in the body for life – so if they have been there in the past, they will be present today. Once comfortably installed in the body they have the potential to drive many other nasty diseases. Their targeting of the brain and immune system explains many symptoms. I suspect it is this group of viruses that are responsible for many cases of post viral CFS/ME. Dr Martin Lerner showed that EBV (also known as HHV4, mono, glandular fever or Epstein Barr virus) was causally involved in 81% of post-viral CFS cases.[2]

improvement. This allows an objective measure of progress. Armin laboratories now offer Elispot testing for EBV, and this is a very useful tool. Again, as the immune system defeats the virus, the level of positivity comes down – this is a very helpful clinical tool.

Treatment

There is too much information to be within the scope of this book. See our book *The Infection Game* for details of regimes and specific antimicrobials.

How to get help

It has taken me decades to realise that I cannot help all the sick people in the world. With Craig's help, together with the wonderful team of Katie Twinn and Carolyn May, we have set up a website, Natural Health Worldwide, that allows any patient to contact any doctor, qualified health practitioner or experienced patient and consult on any symptom or method of treatment. Do see www.naturalhealthworldwide.com for lists of Medical Doctors (18 MDs as of November 2023), Qualified Health Professionals (159 QHPs as of November 2023) and Experienced Patients (37 EPs as of November 2023).There are also lists of laboratories and mobile phlebotomists.

Summary

Diagnosis depends on:

- A high level of clinical suspicion – if you don't look you don't see.
- Good tests and interpretation of such.
- Response to treatment – all diagnosis is hypothesis, which must then be put to the test. However, always remember this may not be the sole cause of symptoms.

Finally, once one infection is established then one must recognise that other microbes are more likely to get into the body, perhaps for the same reasons that the first microbes got in – that is, poor defences. So, the existence of one microbe may indicate that other, as yet unidentified, microbes may also be present. The point here is that it will never be sufficient just to target a particular microbe that has been identified. Improving the defences is as vital a part of attacking microbes as is targeting particular microbes. Having had one debilitating infection, always return to Groundhog Chronic (Appendix 1). You will find Craig and me there too!

There is much scepticism among the medical profession about the existence of such a plethora of chronic infections and the effect they have on human health. I stress, once again, that these chronic infections *do* exist and that tackling them can be the key to recovery for many patients. Do not ignore the possibility of this being the case for you, especially if things aren't improving with all the standard work-up as detailed in this book.

A famous European philosopher well sums up where we are at this moment in time:

> *There are two ways to be fooled. One is to believe what isn't true; the other is to refuse to believe what is true.*
>
> Søren Kierkegaard, Danish philosopher (1813 – 1855)

Do not be fooled either way!

Mathematical interlude from Craig

I have been quite restrained in my mathematical wanderings so far, and so I will allow myself a little meander now. The analysis of false positives and negatives has whetted my appetite. Maths is the 'Joy of the Unexpected' to me. And so here we go with three examples.

1. The chessboard and grains of wheat problem

If a chessboard (eight squares by eight) were to have grains of wheat placed upon each square such that one grain were placed on the first square, two on the second, four on the third, and so on (doubling the number of grains on each subsequent square), how many grains of wheat would be on the chessboard when all 64 squares of the chessboard had had their wheat grains put on them?

The answer is a very large number. In fact, if you summed up all the grains of wheat on the chessboard you would have over 2000 times the entire annual world production of wheat, so, more wheat than has ever been cultivated by humans in history.

This story/problem was first recorded in 1256 by Ibn Khallikan (1211 – 1282), renowned Islamic historian, who compiled the celebrated biographical encyclopaedia of Muslim scholars and important men in Muslim history, *Deaths of Eminent Men and the Sons of the Epoch*.

2. Gabriel's horn (also called Torricelli's trumpet)

This does 'get a bit mathsy' (as my Pure Mathematics Lecturer at Oxford used to say), but take a look at the picture (Figure 20.1) and hopefully all will be clear. Gabriel's horn is the shape you get when you rotate the graph y = 1/x around the x axis between 1 and infinity. There, I said it.

Figure 20.1: Gabriel's horn

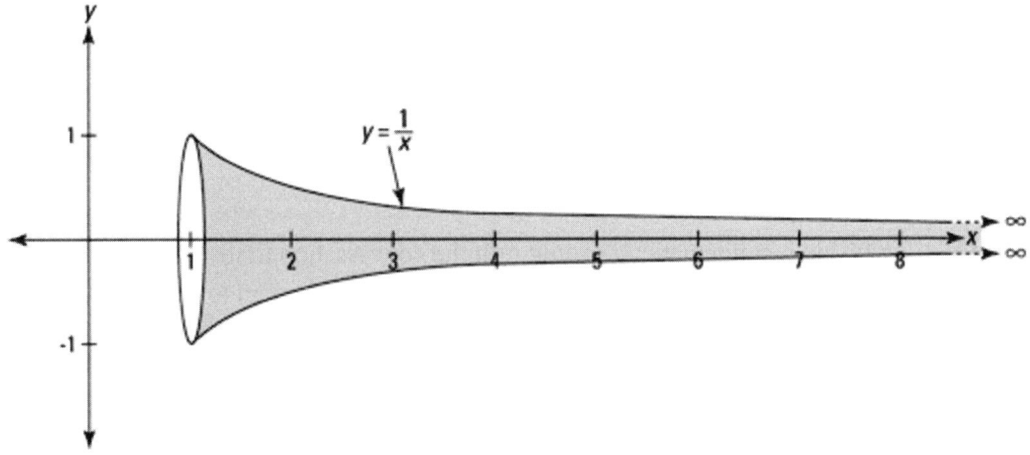

Basically, it's an infinitely long horn that gets quite thin quite soon.

So, what's the unexpected bit then? Well, this horn can be shown to have:

- Finite volume
- Infinite surface area.

Since the horn has finite volume but infinite surface area, there is a paradox in that the horn could be filled with a finite quantity of paint and yet that paint would not be sufficient to coat its surface. In fact, no amount of paint would be enough to coat this horn's surface.

3. Taxicab numbers

Finally, just one of those lovely 'Mathematician Stories' that abound. A little unexpected maybe. There was a marvellous mathematician named Srinivasa Ramanujan‡ FRS (1887 – 1920) who was largely self-taught, growing up in Madras. Some of his (very original) work was passed to various British mathematicians and eventually G H Hardy FRS (English mathematician, 1877 – 1947, author of *A Mathematician's Apology*) realised brilliance when he saw it. Ramanujan was invited over to Cambridge University. For those who are interested, the film *The Man Who Knew Infinity* comes recommended by me. It tells the story with empathy and truth. Anyway, sadly Ramanujan suffered with ill health for most of his life and Hardy recounts: 'I remember once going to see him when he was ill at Putney. I had ridden in taxicab number 1729 and remarked that the number seemed to me rather a dull one, and that I hoped it was not an unfavourable omen. "No," he replied, "it is a very interesting number; it is the smallest number expressible as the sum of two cubes in two different ways."'

First of all, who but a mathematician would turn the conversation to the number of his cab? And then reference the possibility that this might be a bad omen to a sick friend? But, what a reply by the sick Ramanujan! The two sets of cubes he is talking about are:

$1729 = 1^3 + 12^3$ [i.e. = 1 x 1 x 1 PLUS 12 x 12 x 12]
$1729 = 9^3 + 10^3$ [i.e. = 9 x 9 x 9 PLUS 10 x 10 x 10]

This observation (which came from who knows where; Ramanujan‡ credited his mathematical acumen to his family goddess 'Namagiri Thayar', led to a branch of mathematics called 'Taxicab numbers'.

Summary

- If you have put in place all else in this book and you are still ill, then consider the possibility of a chronic infection.
- Diagnose such chronic infection by:
  - Medical history
  - Tests – but be cautious over interpretation
  - Current signs and symptoms.
- Treatment is as per our book *The Infection Game* and/or find yourself a good practitioner from Natural Health Worldwide - https://naturalhealthworldwide.com – or elsewhere.

‡**Postscript:** It is now thought that Ramanujan's health problems were caused by a chronic infection, hepatic amoebiasis. This results from amoebic dysentery, which if not properly treated, can lie dormant for years and eventually lead to hepatic amoebiasis. At the time, if properly diagnosed, amoebiasis was a treatable and often curable disease – many British soldiers contracted it during WWI and many were cured,[3] but the diagnosis was never made in Ramanujan. The doctors thought he had tuberculosis. Ramanujan died aged just 32.

Chapter 21

The emotional holes in the energy bucket

It is beyond my skills and the scope of this book to go into psychological therapies, but there are a few tricks which help. There are some very good psychological therapists who also understand CFS, ME and LC, often via direct personal experience, on Natural Health Worldwide (please see https://naturalhealthworldwide.com and Useful resources on page 303). In addition, Craig has written a webpage – 'Balancing' – which is all about how to balance emotional needs with practical needs, and also the need for recovery. He has written this from an ME sufferer's point of view – see https://drmyhill.co.uk/wiki/Balancing

The Ancients understood how we humans tick:

> *Human behaviour flows from three main sources: desire, emotion and knowledge.*
>
> Plato, Greek philosopher (428/427 or 424/423 BC – 348/347 BC (age c. 80))

You should have the knowledge by now (from reading this book), and I know you will have the desire. So, what about the emotions?

Why more energy will help with the emotional holes

Improving energy delivery mechanisms gives one the energy to employ the psychological tricks of the trade. The brain accounts for 2% of our body weight but consumes 20% of all the energy generated in the body.[1] Michelle E Watts and colleagues (2018) stated that: 'While making up only a small fraction of our total body mass, the brain represents the largest source of energy consumption—accounting for over 20% of total oxygen metabolism. Of this, it is estimated that neurons consume 75%–80% of energy produced in the brain.'[1]

If the brain is constantly busy dealing with past traumas or worrying about the future, then that is hugely wasteful of energy. I do not pretend to be an expert in plugging those emotional holes. These are usually created by a past history of mental, physical, emotional and/or sexual abuse which leaves the sufferer with post-traumatic stress syndrome, hard-wired for hyper-vigilance and insomnia. Doctors compound this by not taking CFS, ME and LC seriously, giving the clear impression that they are dealing with idle hypochondriacs instead of diagnosing real pathology. This rubs off on friends and relations, leaving the sufferer even more isolated.

There can be a reluctance among CFS, ME and LC sufferers to engage with any form of psychological therapy. This can be for many understandable reasons:

- Some wish to concentrate as much effort as possible on the practical and physical core things for facilitating a recovery.
- Some think that attention to emotional needs might give the impression that they are suffering from a psychological illness and that is a battle they don't want to fight again and again.
- For some, the illness has worn them down to such an extent that they have lost a sense of self-value and so actually don't think that 'their' emotional needs are worth attending to.

But addressing the emotional holes can be a very important, indeed actually crucial, stage on the road map, for some, and so please do consider carefully your own individual circumstances. Given all the accumulation of truly awful symptoms and the disbelief from society in general, possibly also from friends and family, and almost certainly from doctors, it would be surprising if there were no emotional holes.

Direct effects of improving energy delivery mechanisms

Improving energy delivery mechanisms can have a *direct* impact on emotional wellbeing. This effect is much reported in Craig and Katie's Facebook group. Many sufferers ask why sometimes they are very weepy and very fatigued at the same time; one possible answer is that ATP is not only the energy molecule but also a neurotransmitter – to be precise, a co-transmitter: other neurotransmitters, such as serotonin, dopamine, GABA and acetylcholine, will not work unless they are accompanied by a molecule of ATP. So, if ATP levels fall precipitously low, then one feels dreadfully fatigued (because of a lack of ATP in its role as the energy molecule) and simultaneously very low emotionally (because of a lack of ATP in its role as co-transmitter). To mitigate this 'double whammy', Craig carries a hip flask of water with 5 grams of D-ribose dissolved in it and this works as a great 'rescue remedy' for when he experiences these sudden ATP dips (thankfully, rarely these days).

Personal note from Craig

Other physiological lesions in CFS, ME and LC sufferers can also have direct effects on emotional wellbeing – for example, adrenal dysfunction can cause anxiety-like symptoms – so addressing these physical lesions can reduce the size of the 'emotional hole'. However, I also found that, simply by addressing the identified physiological problems, a large part of my emotional hole just 'disappeared'. For me, this was because my emotional hole was caused, for the most, by feelings of 'loss' and 'grief' at missing out, and so, as I addressed the physical issues, my functionality improved, and so I could 'join in' more with everyday life and so not miss out so much, thereby reducing the loss and grief 'head on', as it were. This is not to lessen the importance of psychological help – this too can be very helpful, especially if the physical improvements are slow at coming.

Beware of doctors and psychiatrists

We have not moved far since Nicholas Culpepper, a 17th century medical herbalist, stated:

> *Three kinds of people mainly disease the people – priests, physicians and lawyers – priests disease matters belonging to their souls, physicians disease matters belonging to their bodies, and lawyers disease matters belonging to their estate.*
>
> Nicholas Culpepper, English medical herbalist (1616 – 1654)

Doctors do not look for the mechanisms of fatigue and inflammation; they simply wallpaper over the cracks with antidepressants, cognitive behaviour therapy (CBT) and graded exercise therapy (GET). The latter treatment is an oxymoron – for a disease defined by exercise intolerance, this will only make things worse. It is akin to advising the blind to start driving, firemen to dowse flames with petrol and anorexics to restrict calories.

Psychiatrists are past masters at making 'diagnoses' which are not diagnoses at all but simply clinical pictures. These include 'somatisation', 'chronic pain syndrome', 'conversion disorder' (hysteria), 'Munchausen's syndrome' and, in the case of children, 'Munchausen's syndrome by proxy'. I do recommend reading Dr James Davies's book *Cracked: Why Psychiatry is Doing More Harm than Good.*[2] This is a marvellous critique of Western psychiatric practice, which simply funnels patients into drug treatment categories. These categories are laid down by *The Diagnostic and Statistical Manual of Mental Disorders* (DSM), a Big-Pharma-driven production.[3] A lovely analogy Davies draws is with the night sky – psychiatrists are still drawing lines between stars and diagnosing 'Gemini', 'Taurus' and 'Aries'. They are diagnostic flat-Earthers who ignore modern science. We need astronomers using science, not astrologers using the zodiac to diagnose and treat CFS/ME.

So, choose your psychological therapist carefully; the bare minimum is that they *must* know that CFS, ME and LC are physiological illnesses. They must also understand that you are coming to them for help with your emotional holes, and not for a miracle cure, because such a miracle cure simply does not exist.

Having made their 'diagnosis', doctors prescribe medication which is often addictive or inhibits energy-delivery mechanisms. The sufferer gets worse, refuses to take the medication and is labelled as non-compliant. This gives the doctors an excuse to deny them state or other benefits. Many risk a more serious psychiatric diagnosis which may give the psychiatrist powers to take them into a psychiatric unit, against their wishes, under psychiatric 'section'. Beware of doctors! Question them and ask them to give the evidence base for their advice, with real science.

Indeed, much of my job I see as protecting CFS, ME and LC sufferers from the psychiatric profession by establishing the underlying causal physical and pathological mechanisms. And of course, the recent review of the UK's NICE Guideline on ME/CFS [NG206][5] (see Chapter 1) has improved the situation somewhat, by removing GET as a treatment option, for example. But the psychiatrists do not give up that easily, and many CFS and ME sufferers are currently facing being 're-diagnosed' so that the 'old' discredited psychological interventions can be continued under the guise of a newly diagnosed condition. And some LC sufferers are being offered 'music therapy' by the NHS… As important as music is to my life and many others', listening to it will not cure the physiological lesions in LC!

The tricks of the trade for mending the emotional holes

Good quality sleep (see Chapter 8)

Past traumas are dealt with, and dispatched, during non-REM (deep) sleep. Improving sleep quality is therefore very helpful. Simply doing the PK diet irons out blood sugar levels while correcting the underactive thyroid sorts ketogenic hypoglycaemia; with both, there is a flattening of adrenalin spikes. Those ghastly flashbacks which may occur during sleep are then no longer accompanied by the effects of adrenalin and so the brain is able to shut the door and rationalise that particular horror.

Love and be loved

The Beatles knew that love is all we need.

This is where pets are so wonderful. I love my scruffy old Patterdale terrier, Nancy, and we do everything together and look out for each other. She is essential for my psychological welfare. I feel safe at night with her sleeping on my bed and when I go camping. She says this to me every day: 'If you live to be a hundred, I want to live to be a hundred minus one day, so I would never have to live without you' (with thanks to Winnie the Pooh).

The Romans also knew the value of the love of pets, especially their dogs. They buried them and wrote epitaphs. Here are just two examples of many:

> *I am in tears, while carrying you to your last resting place as much as I rejoiced when bringing you home in my own hands fifteen years ago.*
>
> *To Helena, foster child,* soul without comparison and deserving of praise.*

Money helps

It so annoys me when people say 'money does not make you happy'. Nonsense – it don't half help. With money you have security and can buy good food and good care, keep warm and have some energy left over to have fun.

> *I've been rich, and I've been poor. And, believe me, rich is better.*
>
> Attributed to many but perhaps the first 'in-print' attribution was to Beatrice Kaufman who urged a noted theatrical figure to accept the movie offers being tendered to him.[6]

Obtain the state and other benefits to which you are entitled.

***Historical note:** Domestic canines were often referred to as 'foster children' by Romans and that, in itself, sums up how the Romans felt about these life companions.

Much of my time is spent in helping CFS, ME and LC sufferers gain appropriate state and other insurance benefits. This is also an essential part of managing their medical condition since financial security is essential for good emotional health (see Appendix 4, page 269).

Connect with others

CFS, ME and LC can be very isolating, and these feelings of isolation can set up more vicious circles that only worsen the situation. Connecting with others used to be well-nigh impossible for housebound or bedridden CFS and ME sufferers before the advent of the internet and social media. There has been a lot of misinformation written about the negative impact of support groups upon illness outcomes, with some psychiatrists stating that such support groups reinforce 'illness beliefs' and prolong disability. This is not so. Geraghty and colleagues demonstrated this admirably in their paper 'The 'cognitive behavioural model' of chronic fatigue syndrome: Critique of a flawed model'.[4] In any case, the new NICE Guideline [NG206][5] has pooh-poohed the idea of false illness beliefs in CFS and ME:

> *1.12.32 Explain that CBT for people with ME/CFS:*
>
> *--aims to improve their quality of life, including functioning, and reduce the distress associated with having a chronic illness*
>
> *--does not assume people have 'abnormal' illness beliefs and behaviours as an underlying cause of their ME/CFS, but recognises that thoughts, feelings, behaviours and physiology interact with each other.*

Linking with other sufferers can provide a life-line for many people, where not only support and understanding can be found, but sometimes deep friendships develop. This has been the case, I know, for my co-author, Craig, and his Facebook Group co-admin, Katie Twinn, who have developed a special bond, with Craig attending Katie's wedding to Mark in 2017, Katie and Mark spending time in Craig and Penny's caravan in North Norfolk, and then Craig dedicating our book *The Infection Game* to Katie.

One caveat (and again, both Craig and Katie have experienced this) is that time spent on social media can 'fly by' and one can end up using energy that one does not really have. So, as with all things, be careful to pace your time on social media and do factor it into your energy equation. As mentioned in Useful resources (page 303), this list of patient-generated sources of support is a very good starting point: www.drmyhill.co.uk/wiki/CFS/ME_support_organisations.

It is important to recognise that the business of caring requires huge amounts of energy – physical, mental and emotional. The carers need care too. Indeed, caring for a CFS, ME or LC sufferer can be very damaging to relationships because energy flow needs to be a two-way thing, and the CFS, ME or LC sufferer cannot reciprocate in full. This must be recognised and acknowledged with politeness which, at least, is not energy sapping. Saying 'please' and 'thank you' goes a long way. This is in everyone's self-interest and applies equally to carers who are life partners and to carers of any other form – look after your carer! (See the Hammersmith Books' book *Who Cares?*)

Craig and Katie's Facebook groups (see page 204) now have over 18,000 members and are a fabulous source of support and information.

> *A problem shared is a problem halved.*
>
> Old English saying of unknown origin†

†**Literary note:** The first written form of this saying seems to have appeared in the American newspaper, *The Muncie Evening Press*, in November 1854, where the longer form including the phrase 'A joy shared is a joy doubled' was also referenced.

Laughter is the best medicine

Try to have a good sense of humour – laughter really is the best medicine.[‡] If you feel a bit down, click on this link www.youtube.com/watch?v=SJUhlRoBL8M and sing along – I do! Find what amuses you and do it.

Rest and relaxation

If you are very sick, you *have* to rest.

Learn to do meditation. Done well, this can be as restorative as sleep. It helps to make pacing less boring.

Many severe sufferers find the use of heart rate monitoring devices helpful. It is beyond the scope of this book to discuss this topic so please search for 'Heart Rate Monitoring' or 'HRM' online. There are some excellent groups.

At the same time, do *not* do the following:

- Do not try to 'catch up' for those 'lost years'.
- Do not mourn the loss of things not done.
- Do not try to do everything with anyone![§]

[‡]**Literary note:** 'Laughter is the best medicine' is a regular feature in *Reader's Digest* magazine. It consists of medically-based short funny stories or jokes. *Reader's Digest* remains the largest paid-circulation magazine in the world (global circulation of 10.5 million as of November 2023) and was 100 years old on 5 February 2022. Craig used to read this section, and a few others, on visits to his grandfather. It became a tradition to see Craig sitting in the corner chuckling away at some joke or another. He was allowed to tear out the 'Increase your Word Power' sections and take them home with him.

[§]**Personal note by Craig:** I have read *The Great Gatsby* (by F Scott Fitzgerald,[¶] American author, 1896 – 1940) more times than is good for one's health. I am often heard quoting from it: 'I wish I had done everything on Earth with you' (from the screenplay, not the book.)

Instead, celebrate each milestone and, like Gatsby, 'believe in the green light' but not as some unobtainable, unrequited lost love or experience, but rather as an horizon, something always to aim for and always to look forward to. Be resolute in all the physiological interventions described in this book. Keep going and never ever give up! As the Gallagher brothers said so well: 'Don't look back in anger', or at least if you do, recognise what you are doing and banish those thoughts as quickly as you can.

¶**Self-reflection by Craig:** F Scott Fitzgerald is amongst my favourite authors, and I often used to wonder why. So, I did a little research, and it turns out that many people think he had synaesthesia, as do I, and that many synaesthetics also love his work. It is thought that this is the case because he writes 'synaesthetically' – that is, using descriptive passages that 'mix up' the senses – and that this appeals to synaesthetics because he is 'using their language'.[7, 8] Fitzgerald uses these synaesthetic-type phrases, especially in *The Great Gatsby*. Teri Floyd[8] in the article 'Your name tastes like purple' says that she has read Gatsby many times and that it never bores her because of the perpetual flow of colour throughout the book. For my part, the most eloquent three-word description of any party occurs in *The Great Gatsby*: it is described as having 'yellow cocktail music'.

Summary

- Having CFS, ME or LC is *tough* – tougher than most people will ever know. It would be surprising if sufferers did *not* have an emotional hole.
- Do all the physiological interventions because this will help to minimise the psychological impact, both directly and indirectly.
- Overcome the reluctance you may feel to engage with psychological interventions. Do analyse yourself and decide whether such interventions might be helpful to your recovery.
- Choose your psychological therapist very carefully, paying attention to *their* beliefs. They must know that CFS, ME and LC are physiological illnesses.
- Get good quality sleep.
- Love and be loved – get a pet if you can. (Craig can't – he is so allergic. But he has Penny!)
- Maximise your money (legally!).
- Connect with other sufferers.
- Take care of your carers.
- Try to allow your sense of humour to show.
- For the very sick, these things may not be possible – meditation and other mindfulness techniques can help to maximise rest and to close that emotional hole too.

Chapter 22

The pattern of recovery

The general principles are:

- Recovery is like building a house – start with the foundations (PK diet and the Basic Package of supplements) and keep building. Craig has written a webpage which models why the foundations are so important: 'Chaos Theory and CFS/ME recovery paths' – see www.drmyhill.co.uk/wiki/Chaos_Theory_and_CFS/ME_recovery_paths. In architecture, we understand the importance of solid foundations, so much so that important buildings often have a 'Foundation(al) stone' laid by an important dignitary.*
- Do not give up on an earlier step because you have not seen a clinical benefit.
- As you get older you will have to work harder at it.
- Expect a bumpy ride (see Appendix 2: DDD reactions).
- Whilst you are improving and continuing to improve, carry on.

***Foundation(al) stones:** These are stones laid with some public ceremony to denote the completion of a large, important building. And the phrase 'foundation stone' has come to mean a basic principle upon which all else relies. Here are two examples of foundation stones:

1. King's College Chapel, Cambridge – In 1446, during the Feast of St James, and shortly before the Wars of the Roses, King Henry VI laid the foundation stone of this chapel, a chapel that was intended to be a small part of a greater court. Though the court was never completed, the chapel still stands, complete with foundation stone.
2. The mysterious 'London Stone' – Time has all but erased the history of the London Stone, although it is believed to be of Roman origin, and its name can be traced back to the 1100s. This chunk of limestone is a small portion of the original piece once secured into the ground. It was moved in 1742 and was built into the south wall of the Church of St Swithun London Stone in 1798. Though the church was demolished in the 1960s, the stone remains.

- At the point at which you plateau or get stuck, introduce a new intervention. Re-read this book!
- Always start new interventions with low doses and build up slowly. The sicker you are, the more important this is.
- Do not rely on others, least of all doctors. The majority are obstructive and prescribe drugs which may buy you a window of relief for a time but will slow eventual recovery.

Use your brain think ahead:

- The most powerful triggers to a relapse are infection and vaccines.
- Make sure your first aid box is stocked with the necessary tools so you can immediately act at first hint of any infection (see Appendix 1: Groundhog Acute).
- Do not vaccinate. The Covid mRNA gene therapy 'vaccines' have proved ineffective and dangerous.
- Choose where you take your holidays wisely.
- There is much more detail in our books *Ecological Medicine* and *The Infection Game* for those who need convincing.

Non-linear recovery with catastrophic events

The pattern of recovery will not be linear, and it will not be monotonic – see Figure 22.1, which models how recovery happens. Monotonic is a word much used in mathematics; in essence it describes a pattern of behaviour that always 'moves in the same direction'.

We start life in the top left-hand corner of Figure 22.1 (point X). Unhealthy lifestyles erode our wellbeing, and we gradually slide down the slippery slope. Then there may be a catastrophic trigger, at point A: viral infection, poisoning, bereavement, trauma, financial crisis or whatever. We drop off the edge of the curve, landing at point A', and eventually, we may slide to the bottom right-hand corner (point Y).

The journey back to the top left-hand corner health is much more difficult. It is a hard slog up the slippery slope. But suddenly you get to that critical point, B, all is in place, the brain and body can safely come out of Naviaux's defensive hibernation mode and energy is available with which to have a life, and you flip up the curve to B'. Welcome back to the world!

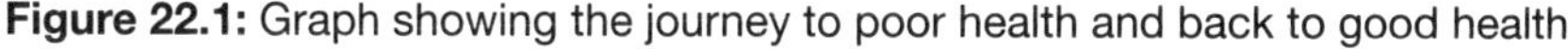

Figure 22.1: Graph showing the journey to poor health and back to good health

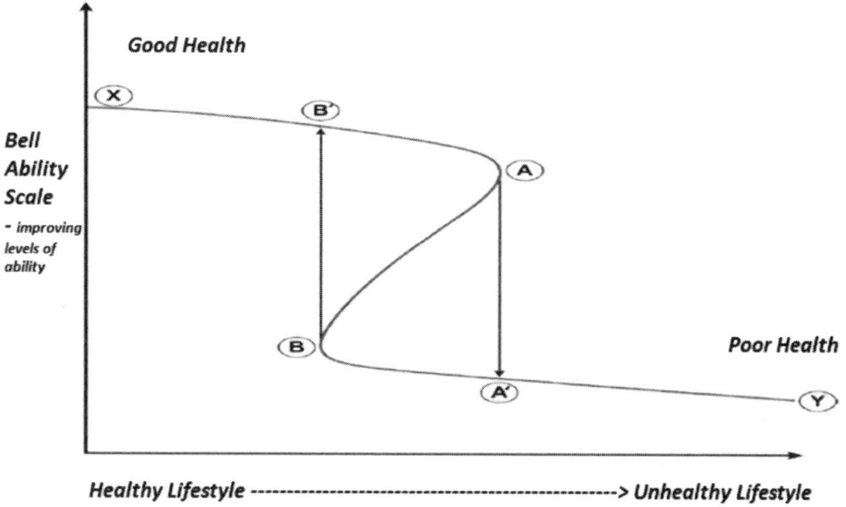

I have witnessed some remarkable recovery stories in my four decades of medical practice. Think of Craig not being able to count from one to 10 and then helping with my books and website and writing his varying maths problems book.

Recently, one of my secretaries received an email, asking that it be passed onto me. It read thus:

> *C……. could you mention this to Sarah when you communicate next?*
>
> *I would just like her to know that after reading her book (advertised within a website article) my life turned around. Having ME since childhood I was diagnosed in 1984 as having ME. Since then, all the help and remedies, even*

from the ME support magazines, dealt only with the symptoms. Seemingly in their research, the 'experts' were acting on individual symptoms as causes. On reading your ME book I found you listed 100% of my symptoms and gave me the root cause of the ME and guidance to managing and healing from ME, which WORKED! I am functioning near 'normally' now and always recommend your work widely to other ME sufferers. THANK YOU so much for the work you do and also my ability to function not only well, but better than some others 'of my age group' around me!

This person had run 50 miles in just over nine hours, up and down the Shropshire Hills, and had come third out of a large field of very fit competitors. So, dear reader… now comes some very important advice…

Never, ever give up

The poster below used to be pinned outside my consulting room and its words have become the Group Motto of the Facebook Group – 'Support for Followers of Dr Myhill's Porotcol' (see Useful resources, page 303).

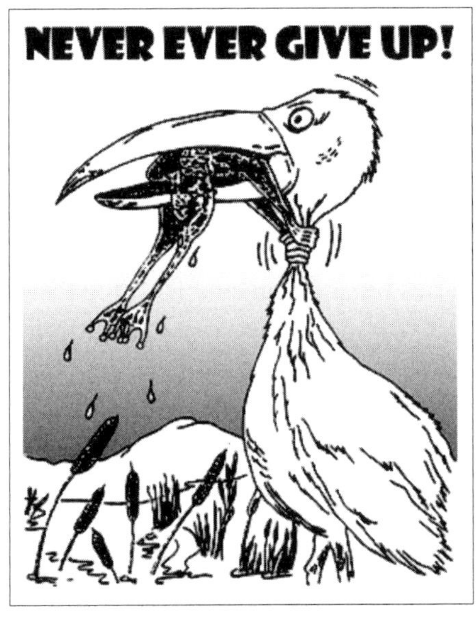

The words of Sir Winston Churchill (30 November 1874 – 24 January 1965) echo in my ears:

> *Never give in. Never give in. Never, never, never, never—in nothing, great or small, large or petty—never give in, except to convictions of honour and good sense. Never yield to force. Never yield to the apparently overwhelming might of the enemy.*

The enemy here is CFS, ME or LC.

Whoever you take your inspiration from, never ever give in. That point 'B' could be just round the corner, and, as Craig has said, there are good times ahead of you, waiting for you to be there.

Summary

- Get the foundation stones in place and keep them in place – the PK diet and the Basic Package.
- Keep on with the road map, even in the face of no (quick) improvements.
- When something works, carry on doing it.
- Expect things to be bumpy – very bumpy at times.
- Try new interventions to move things forward, but always start low and slow.
- Use your brain to avoid catastrophic events – see above.
- Crucially, never ever give up.

Chapter 23

The politics of CFS and ME

The name, the shame and the blame

In politics, stupidity is not a handicap.

Napoleon Bonaparte (1769 – 1821), de facto leader of the French Republic as First Consul from 1799 to 1804, then Emperor of the French from 1804 until 1814, and again in 1815

Reader, suppose you were an idiot. And suppose you were a member of Congress. But I repeat myself.

Mark Twain (1835 – 1910), American writer, humourist, entrepreneur, publisher and lecturer

The name: when the name masquerades as a diagnosis

The practice of medicine used to be an honourable occupation practised by doctors who listened to patients, catalogued their symptoms and tried to work out the mechanisms behind what was going on. Having established the cause there were clear implications for treatment. This is called diagnosis – with the mechanism established, the treatment followed naturally and logically. In the treatment of chronic conditions, doctors no longer diagnose. They no longer work out mechanisms. Yes – it is laughable.*

***Joke:** How did the mathematician cure his constipation? He worked it out with a pencil.

Doctors may be good at recognising and giving names to clinical pictures, but this now masquerades as a diagnosis. The clinical picture of chronic fatigue is variously recognised under the name of 'yuppie 'flu', 'myalgic encephalomyelitis', 'post-viral syndrome', 'Royal Free syndrome', 'systemic exertion intolerance disease' (SEID), 'chronic fatigue immune dysfunction syndrome' (CFIDS) and many others. Quite naturally and understandably patients assume, once their illness has been named, that appropriate treatment which will address the causes will follow. Wrong!

Conventional medicine offers a package of treatments none of which bears any resemblance to causation. Worse, symptom-suppressing medication accelerates the underlying pathology and patients are made worse. Temporary mood enhancers, such as Prozac, render sufferers emotionally numb but do nothing for energy-delivery mechanisms. They leave the patient addicted and are a risk factor for suicide. We have been left with this intellectually risible situation because Big Pharma educates doctors who then cow-tow. More drugs mean more side effects which mean more drugs. Great for Big Pharma profits. Remember its mantra: 'A patient cured is a customer lost.'

The blame

CFS and ME have many causes and triggers, many of which are due to bad practice and false assurances. These gradually erode health and then just one 'extra' cause (e.g. acute Covid-19) may suffice as a trigger. My view is that, in order of importance (Table 23.1), these cheap-skating practices are the most to blame. (Once again, this book is not a textbook, and so I will provide some references or at least links to places where you can go, if interested in the detail.)

Table 23.1: The factors that lead to chronic fatigue

What	**Why**	**Sources and references**
Fast foods	High-carb addictive foods driving diabetes and obesity Micronutrient deficient Food additives (3500 chemical can be legally added to foods) – the more a food is processed the greater its toxicity	See our book *Paleo-Ketogenic: The Why and the How* for much more detail. See Chapter 4 of this book
Addictions	Smoking, vaping, alcohol, caffeine etc	The risks of smoking and alcohol consumption are well documented but there is growing evidence about the risks of vaping also[1, 2, 3]
Big Pharma	Experimental gene therapy mRNA 'vaccines' – there have been more side effects from these than all other vaccinations administered in the history of vaccines	VAERS is the Vaccine Adverse Event Reporting Scheme operating in the US. OpenVAERS allows browsing and searching of the VAERS reports without the need to compose an advanced search. The most recent update as of going to print (at September 2023) stated these figures for the Covid-19 vaccine: 1,596,983 adverse events, 36,324 deaths, 210,347 hospitalisations.[4a] For children, the data show (also as at September 2023) 67,893 adverse events, 189 deaths, 5600 hospitalisations, 630 permanently disabled, 10,977 not recovered from adverse event.[4b] In the UK, via the Yellow Card Reporting System (which undoubtedly misses many adverse events), we have (as at February 2023) from the UK Freedom Project: 1,642,357 adverse events and 2459 deaths.[4c] For readers who wish to look at the data in more detail, please see Dr Mark Trozzi's excellent website, with more than 1000 peer-reviewed articles on vaccine injuries.[4d] https://drtrozzi.org/2023/09/28/1000-peer-reviewed-articles-on-vaccine-injuries/
	Other vaccines: nanoparticle metals, mercury, aluminium	See Chapter 13 plus the article by Gregory and colleagues[5]
	HIV (from polio vaccine) XMRV (from vaccines)	If you have the energy and money buy and read: *The River* by Edward Hooper[6] *Plague* Judy Mikovits[7]

What	Why	Sources and references
	Symptom-suppressing drugs	See our book *Ecological Medicine*
	Silicone implants	
Big Farma	Herbicides and pesticides in food, spray drift, garden poisons, insect control	If you have the energy and money buy and read *Toxic Legacy* by Stephanie Seneff[8]
Manu-facturing industry	Discharge heavy metals, volatile organic compounds and pesticides into air and water. Small particulate matter	See the work of Dr Dick van Steenis[9] and the contribution by van Steenis to the *House of Commons Environmental Audit Committee Air quality: A follow up report Ninth Report of Session 2010–12*[10]
Dentists	Dental amalgam	See my web page[11]
Building industry	Sick building syndrome	If you have the energy and money buy and read *Chemical Sensitivity – low levels, high stakes* by Claudia Miller[12]
	Damp with fungi and mycotoxins	See Lisa Petrison's website https://paradigmchange.me/lisa/ Free download pdf books available
	Carbon monoxide poisoning	See the 2002 article by J Wright[13]
Internal decorations	Carpet and paint solvents Fire retardants (polybrominated biphenyls poison us in parts per trillion – that is one drop in an Olympic-size pool)	If you have the energy and money buy and read *Chemical Sensitivity – low levels, high stakes* by Claudia Miller[12]
Air pollution from vehicles	Diesel particulates, nitrogen compounds, ozone, petrol additives	See the work of Dr Dick van Steenis[9, 10]
Aeroplanes	Organophosphates	Aerotoxic syndrome – see https://aerotoxic.org Free download pdf books available

Table 23.1 *Cont'd*

What	Why	Sources and references
All of us	Microplastics (MPs) Human excrement which is not composted but pollutes rivers	See the article by Simul Bhuyan (2022) which concluded that: 'Exposure to MPs has also been linked to oxidative stress, cytotoxicity, ….' and '… exposure to MPs for an extended period, potentially leading to chronic discomfort, swelling, cell growth, and death, as well as immune cell impairment. Inflammatory bowel disease was significantly higher in patients with MPs than the healthy people. MPs decreased the growth of Caco-2 cells over time. The mitochondrial membrane potential was disturbed by MPs. MPs may also serve as vectors for a variety of microbes.[14]
Warfare	Biological weapons: • Mycoplasma incognito (released during the Gulf War) • Sars Covid-19 (released from Wuhan labs) • Lyme disease (released from Fort Detrick)	If you have the energy and money buy and read *Bitten* by Kris Newby.[15] (Note from Craig: Sarah gave me a copy of this (and also of *The River*, as above) – they are both excellent treatises on their chosen subjects)
Radiation leaks	Chernobyl, Fukushima Testing of nuclear weapons	The ill effects are well known and documented
FINALLY Acute viral infections	All the above suppress the immune system. Aim to do Groundhog Chronic. Be prepared to do Groundhog Acute	See our book *The Infection Game* See Appendix 1.

What is common to many of the above conditions is that there have been huge patient-driven campaigns to recognise these syndromes so that appropriate litigation and compensation can follow. I have often been involved. The outcome is predictable – the Establishment ignore, deny and bury the issue to ensure a cheap conclusion. Where, in individual cases, compensation has resulted, a gagging clause has been applied so that no others can follow that route.

The shame – when the Truth is buried

To achieve the above, successive Governments have colluded with doctors to bury proper recognition of CFS, ME, and now LC, and continue to run with clinical pictures that pander to the different pressure groups. A network of consultant psychiatrists have received millions of pounds of government and industry money to establish chronic fatigue syndrome (CFS) as a psychiatric disorder. This process of obfuscating the truth culminated in the so-called PACE trial 2011,[16] which cost in the region of £5million. This trial has now been shown to be a national disgrace.

The PACE study and what happened after it was published

In summary, the PACE study claimed to be a randomised controlled trial (the gold-standard of research methods if followed correctly) that assessed adaptive pacing (APT), cognitive behaviour therapy (CBT) and graded exercise therapy (GET) as safe and effective treatments for CFS. The authors of the study concluded that, when added to standard medical care (SMC), CBT and GET had greater success in reducing fatigue and improving physical function than did SMC alone. They reported that 22% of patients in the CBT and GET groups had recovered following these therapies, compared with 8% in the APT and 7% in the SMC-only group. In order to understand these conclusions, one needs to know what those acronyms mean:

SMC (specialist medical care): This consisted of medication for symptoms such as insomnia and pain, and general advice to avoid extremes of rest and inactivity.

CBT (cognitive behavioural therapy): In the PACE trial this therapy focused on addressing the presumed fear of activity that the PACE authors thought CFS sufferers had. CBT in general terms is a talking therapy that can help you manage your disease or disorder by changing the way you think and behave.

GET (graded exercise therapy): For this trial, this therapy focused on increasing physical activity in a structured manner, with regular aerobic exercise as the eventual goal. GET calls for these increases in activity despite any increasing fatigue or pain.

APT (adaptive pacing therapy): This is what we have referred to as 'Pacing' in this book. Patients manage their activity levels within their energy envelopes.

Published in the prestigious journal, *The Lancet*, this paper became the internationally recognised basis for 'best practice' in treating CFS, resulting in many patients becoming much more ill as they struggled to fulfil the exercise regimes or were refused state benefits because of 'non-compliance'.

Patients and proper doctors knew that GET made people worse and so applied to see the raw data upon which the authors of the research had relied. This was refused and a court action ensued headed by Alem Matthees, an ME/CFS advocate who lives with very severe ME (see https://me-pedia.org/wiki/Alem_Matthees). The PACE authors used another £200,000 of public monies to resist, but were refused and The First Tier Tribunal ordered the release of the data.[17, 18]

The raw data were then properly analysed by an authoritative statistician and doctor, namely Keith Geraghty. He came to very different conclusions to those of the PACE trial authors. He found that actually, the treatments were not only ineffective but made things worse. His published paper was sent to the PACE authors for comment. Then all three documents were passed to 40 independent academics around the world for publication in the *Journal of Health Psychology*. Those 40 academics agreed with Geraghty and so eager were they to put the record straight that one comment included: 'I will get these data off my computer directly on my return to the office and shall start work on this immediately'. And indeed, these 40 other academics did get the raw data from their computers and began looking at it in detail. Other critiques were made, more flaws were uncovered, and all were included in a 'Special Edition' of the Journal.[19]

Letters to the Editor of *The Lancet*, where the PACE trial was published, ensued, calling for its retraction. No such retraction has come. David Tuller, Senior Fellow in Public Health in Journalism at the Center of Global Public Health, took on the task of galvanising doctors and scientists from around the world, and three open letters were published and were signed by hundreds of eminent doctors and scientists.[20, 21, 22]

These letters pointed out the very serious errors made in that PACE trial, for example, and these two points are only representative:

Point 1: Serious disability was defined as recovery

> The Lancet *paper included an analysis in which the outcome thresholds for being within the normal range on the two primary measures of fatigue and physical function demonstrated worse health than the criteria for entry, which already indicated serious disability. In fact, 13 per cent of the study participants were already within the normal range on one or both outcome measures at baseline, but the investigators did not disclose this salient fact in the* Lancet *paper. In an accompanying* Lancet *commentary, colleagues of the PACE team defined participants who met these expansive normal ranges as having achieved a strict criterion for recovery. The PACE authors reviewed this commentary before publication.*

Point 2: The goalposts were moved

As a result of the PACE authors' actions as described immediately below, participants could end up with worse health measures than the criteria for entry for the trial (serious disability) and still be counted as having improved!

> *Mid-trial, the PACE investigators changed their protocol methods of assessing their primary outcome measures of fatigue and physical function. This is of particular concern in an unblinded trial like PACE, in which outcome trends are often apparent long before outcome data are seen. The investigators provided no sensitivity analyses to assess the impact of the changes and have refused requests to provide the results per the methods outlined in their protocol.*

The PACE authors lowered the bar for 'improvement' midway through the trial because it became evident that participants were not improving!

These errors are so egregious that Colombia University, USA, now uses the PACE Trial as an example of how **not** to design and carry out medical trials.

PACE is intellectual, scientific and financial fraud

In January 2018 I reported the PACE authors to the General Medical Council for multiple breaches of research ethics and Good Medical Practice. It took the GMC six months to refuse to investigate these fraudulent doctors. I requested the evidence base for the GMC's refusal to investigate these offenders and initially the Information Commissioner agreed with me (September 2020) that this evidence base should be disclosed. However, the GMC appealed on the grounds that to release such evidence (and of course you and I know it had nonesuch) would be a tacit admission that the PACE authors were being investigated and this would amount to a breach of their personal right to a private life. A further ICO hearing was a split decision – one member agreed with me, but I lost.

The problem now is that any old doctor can do any old research, which may well be a complete pack of lies, and get away with it. It also means that the GMC can suspend any doctor it likes for any reason that it likes. And it does.

Good doctors are hounded out

Doctors who practise outside the narrow confines of Big-Pharma-driven medicine soon feel the chill wind of Establishment opprobrium. Many have been subject to General Medical Council (GMC) investigations for the same reasons I have as described next: their use of treatments outside of conventional guidelines. They, like me, were trying to diagnose properly, establish underlying mechanisms and treat patients with natural therapies. They include Dr Sam White, Dr Jayne Donegan, Dr Anne McCloskey, Dr Almas U Din Qazi, Dr Julia Piper, Dr David Cartland and many others.

I spent 20 years in unblemished NHS practice. Within a few months of independent practice specialising in the treatment of CFS and ME, I received the first broadside from the Establishment. These have continued since. I am now the most investigated doctor in the history of the GMC. Since 2001 I have been subject to 43 separate investigations by the GMC, involving nine GMC hearings. All these complaints had come either from other doctors or from the GMC itself – not a single patient had complained about my practice (bless them all!). Accusations ranged from recommending nutritional supplements and vitamin B12 injections to the use of the thyroid hormones, the development of mitochondrial function tests and recommendations for using vitamins C and D and iodine. The only accusation of which I was really proud was the accusation that I had brought the reputation of the medical profession into disrepute!

I made very extensive Data Protection Act searches of my GMC records and still the most astonishing comment I have ever seen was this: 'My main concerns with all the Myhill files are that all of the patients appear to be improving and none of them are likely to give WS [witness statements] or have complained about their treatment.' (Mr Tom Kark QC in Internal GMC memo dated 10th February 2006)

I went into independent medicine simply because I did not have the intellectual freedom to be an effective doctor within the NHS. This was a bad move financially – doctors within the NHS are paid regardless of success or ability. So long as they practise tick-box medicine they will be assured a regular salary, sick pay, holiday pay and early retirement with a good pension. No wonder NHS morale is at an all-time low. I discovered that last year 10,000 doctors deregistered from the GMC. I am not the only one!

I have now spent over four decades trying to re-educate the medical profession. I have failed miserably. I realise that in asking them to diagnose and treat CFS, ME and now LC correctly, I am asking them to rethink the whole of their medical practice. This is not just an intellectual revolution for these doctors but also potentially a complete financial

[†]**Joke:** Yes – I know the Ark is a myth but it leads to a good joke. The animals came in two by two including the zebras. Zebra one was looking happy, indeed smug; zebra two was surly and fed up. 'What on earth is wrong with you?' declared Noah. 'You are one of the lucky ones'. Zebra two replied, 'It's not fair… I have both the tapeworms!'

Final note from Craig: I have some choice 16th Century English words about the PACE authors. Here they are:

- Bayard – one with the self confidence that comes with ignorance.
- Mumpsimus – someone who sticks to their opinion even when it's been shown to be wrong.

And if any doctor suggests GET to you, please just quote Hamlet, Act III, Scene III line 87 back at them, namely: 'No!' (https://myshakespeare.com/hamlet/act-3-scene-3)

disaster for them personally. I also realise that this must be a grass-roots revolution. The idea of this book is to wrest power away from the professional doctors and teach the 'amateur' patients to do it for themselves. To that end, this book provides them with the Rules of the Game and the Tools of the Trade to allow each and all to take control of their disease and walk their own path to recovery. Just remember, the Titanic was built by professionals, but amateurs built the Ark.[†]

Summary

- CFS, ME and, as we are already seeing, LC are the worst treated illnesses.
- Doctors use manifestly ineffective, and sometimes downright harmful, treatments, and then blame the patients when they don't recover.
- The Medical Establishment investigates, prosecutes and victimises those doctors who do actually try to treat CFS, ME and LC properly and to good effect.
- Patients must cure themselves, sometimes with the help of good health practitioners.
- This book gives patients the Rules of the Game and the Tools of the Trade with which to affect this recovery.

APPENDICES

Appendix 1

The Groundhog regimes

Because I constantly refer back to the basic approach outlined in this Appendix, which is fundamental to the treatment of all infections, and by inference to the avoidance of the major killers (cancer, heart disease, dementia) which are all now known to be driven by chronic infection, I call them the Groundhogs. In the film *Groundhog Day* the protagonist is caught in a time loop where the same day is repeated again and again until there is a shift in his understanding; my Groundhog regimes represent another sort of loop that bears constant repetition. The point here is that the Groundhogs done well will do much to prevent acute illness developing and chronic disease getting a foothold.

It is also the case that the Groundhogs will change through life as we are exposed to new infections and as our defences decline with age. The key principles are:

- All should do Groundhog Basic all (well, most) of the time.
- All should be prepared to upgrade to Groundhog Acute (page 235) to deal with unexpected and sudden infectious challenges – get that First Aid box stocked up now (page 238)!
- We will all need to move to Groundhog Chronic as we age and acquire an infectious load (page 240).

In summary. we use the Groundhogs like this:

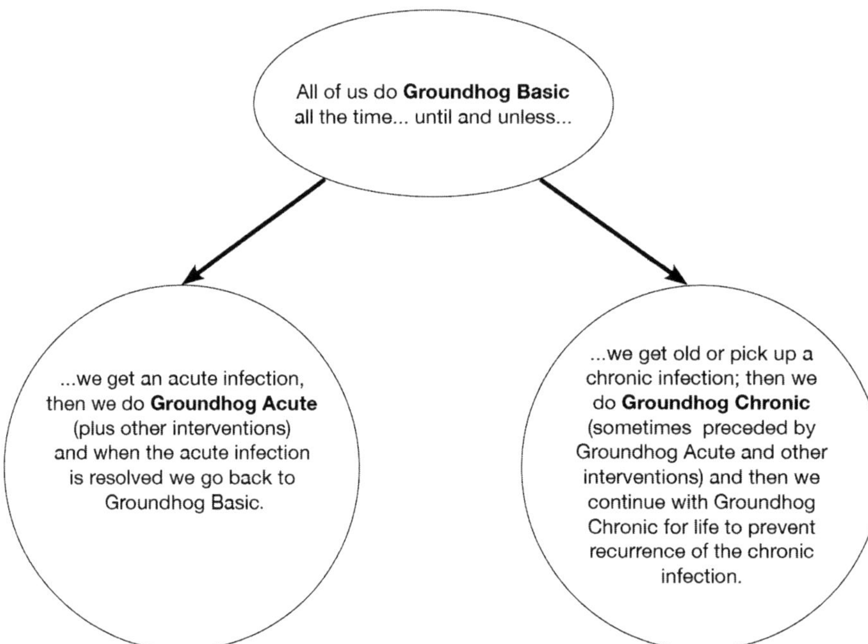

Groundhog Basic

The supplements noted in Table A1.1 are what I call the 'basic package' – they are what we should all be doing all the time, especially the kids.

Table A1.1: Groundhog Basic

What to do	**Notes**
The Paleo-Ketogenic diet: • high fat, high fibre, very low carb • probiotic foods like kefir and sauerkraut • no dairy or grains • two to three meals a day with no snacking	See Chapter 4 and, for more detail, our book *Paleo-Ketogenic: The Why and the How*
A basic package of nutritional supplements – multi-vitamins, multi-minerals, essential fatty acids and vitamin D 10,000 iu	A good multi-vitamin and Sunshine salt 1 tspn daily with food. 1 dsp hemp oil
Vitamin C	Take vitamin C 5 g (or to bowel tolerance levels) little and often through the day; I suggest 1 tsp of ascorbic acid (this will deliver 5 g)
Sleep 8-9 hours between 10:00 pm and 7:00 am	More in winter, less in summer
Exercise at least once a week when you push yourself to your limit (see Chapter 9 for the right sort)	It is anaerobic exercise that produces lactic acid and stimulates the development of new muscle fibres and new mitochondria
Check your breathing (see Chapter 6)	Breathe through your nose, with your diaphragm, and slowly
Herbs, spices and fungi in cooking	Use your favourite herbs, spices and fungi in cooking and food, and lots of them – Yum yum!
If fatigue is an issue - address energy delivery mechanisms as best as you can	Energy delivery mechanisms are addressed in *Ecological Medicine, The Energy Equation* and this book (Chapter 3)

Table A1.1 *Cont'd*

What to do	Notes
Heat and light	Keep warm; sunbathe at every opportunity
Use your brain	Foresight: Avoid risky actions like kissing,* unprotected sex. Caution: Avoid vaccinations; travel with care Circumspection: Do not suppress symptoms with drugs; treat breaches of the skin seriously

Pregnant and breastfeeding women and children

All Groundhog regimes are safe, indeed desirable, for pregnant and breastfeeding women. Children under the age of 12 should halve doses of supplements and take a 'children's multivitamin' such as Biocare Complete Children's Multinutrient; they should work out their own bowel tolerance of vitamin C, just as adults do, but by taking 1 gram/5 grams of vitamin C every hour for Groundhog Basic and Chronic/Groundhog Acute respectively.

It is so important to have all the above in place and then at the first sign of any infection take vitamin C to bowel tolerance and use iodine for local infections, because:

- You will feel much better very quickly.
- Your immune system will not be so activated that it cannot turn off subsequently. So many patients I see with ME started their illness with an acute infection from which they never recovered – their immune system stayed switched on.
- The shorter and less severe the acute infection, the smaller the chance of switching on an inappropriate immune reaction, such as autoimmunity.
- The shorter and less severe the acute infection, the smaller the chance the microbe concerned has of making itself a permanent home in your body. Many diseases, from Crohn's and cancer to polymyalgia and Parkinson's, have an infectious driver (see our book *The Infection Game: Life is an arms race*).

*Oscar Wilde (16 October 1854 – 30 November 1900) knew this, perhaps for different reasons than the risk of infection, when he wrote that: 'A kiss may ruin a human life.' (From *A Woman of No Importance* (is there ever such a thing? asks Craig))

Groundhog Acute – what we should all do at the first sign of any infection, no matter what or where

At the first sign of any infection, you must immediately put in place Groundhog Acute. Do not forget the wise advice of Dr Fred Klenner (BS, MS, MD, FCCP, FAAFP, 1907 – 1984): 'The patient should get large doses of vitamin C in all pathological conditions while the physician ponders the diagnosis.' Strike soon and strike hard because time is of the essence. I repeat myself here because it is so important:

- You will feel much better very quickly.
- Your immune system will not be so activated that it cannot turn off subsequently. So many patients I see with ME started their illness with an acute infection from which they never recovered – their immune system stayed switched on.
- The shorter and less severe the acute infection, the smaller the chance of switching on an inappropriate immune reaction, such as autoimmunity. Many viruses are associated with one type or another of arthritis – for example, 'palindromic rheumatism'[†]. I think of this as viral allergy.
- The shorter and less severe the acute infection, the smaller the chance the microbe concerned has of making itself a permanent home in your body. Many diseases, from Crohn's and cancer to polymyalgia and Parkinson's, have an infectious driver (see our book *The Infection Game*).

At the first sign of the tingling, sore throat, runny nose, malaise, headache, cystitis, skin inflammation, insect bite, or whatever… Table A1.2 shows what you should do.

[†]**Note:** Palindromic rheumatism is rheumatism that comes and goes. The word 'palindrome' was coined by English playwright Ben Johnson in the 17th Century from the Greek roots *palin* (πάλιν: 'again') and *dromos* (δρόμος; 'way, direction'). The first known palindrome, written as a graffito, and etched into the walls of a house in Herculaneum, reads thus: *'sator arepo tenet opera rotas'* – 'The sower Arepo leads with his hand the plough'. (idiomatic translation). Much of the graffiti (graffito is the singular of graffiti) found in Pompeii and Herculaneum are somewhat bawdy, some focusing on what the local ladies of the fine houses would like to do with certain named gladiators or, indeed, vice-versa… The authors leave it to the readers to do their own research.

Table A1.2: Groundhog Acute

What to do	Why and how
The paleo-ketogenic (PK) diet: • high fat, high fibre, very low carb • probiotic foods like kefir and sauerkraut • no dairy or grains • two meals a day; no snacking	See Chapter 4 and our book *Paleo-Ketogenic: The Why and the How*
You may consider a fast – this is essential for any acute gut infection. Drink rehydrating fluids – that is, Sunshine salt 5 g in 1 litre of water ad lib	'Starve a cold; starve a fever' (No, not a typo – starve *any* short-lived infection) (See our book *Paleo-Ketogenic: The Why and the How*)
Vitamin C to bowel tolerance as described in Chapter 4. The need for vitamin C increases hugely with any infection. Interestingly our bowel tolerance changes so one needs a much higher dose to get a loose bowel motion during an infection. If you do not have a very loose bowel motion within one hour of taking 10 g, take another 10 g. Keep repeating until you get to bowel tolerance	As explained in greater detail in Chapter 4, vitamin C greatly reduces any viral, or indeed any microbial, load in the gut (be aware that some of the infecting load of influenza virus will get stuck onto the sticky mucus which lines the lungs and is coughed up and swallowed) Vitamin C improves the acid bath of the stomach. Vitamin C protects us from the inevitable free-radical damage of an active immune system
A good multi-vitamin Sunshine salt 1 tsp daily in water 1 dsp hemp oil	Sunshine salt in water at a ratio of 5 g (1 tsp) in 1 l water to provide a 0.5% solution
Take Lugol's iodine 15%: 2 drops in a small glass of water every hour until symptoms resolve. Swill it round your mouth, gargle, sniff and inhale the vapour. When swilling and gargling, spit out afterwards. The spitting out avoids any possible issues with vitamin C (being a reducing agent) and iodine (being an oxidising agent) 'cancelling each other out'. Sniffing and inhaling iodine will not cancel out vitamin C in the gut because the gut is a different 'department' of the body from the nasal passages	It is well documented that 30 seconds of direct contact with iodine kills all microbes at 10 parts per million, i.e. 0.001%. If you can smell the iodine then you have a therapeutic dose

What to do	Why and how
With respiratory symptoms, put 4 drops of Lugol's iodine 15% into a salt pipe and inhale for 2 minutes; do this at least four times a day. Apply a smear of iodine ointment inside the nostrils (see Useful resources for Providone Iodine Ointment)	As above, 30 seconds of direct contact with iodine kills all microbes. This will contact-kill microbes on their way in or on their way out, rendering you less infectious to others
Apply iodine ointment 10% to any bite, skin break or swelling (see Useful resources for Providone Iodine Ointment)	Again, iodine contact-kills all microbes and is absorbed through the skin to kill invaders
Consume plenty of herbs, spices and fungi	If you are still struggling, then see *The Infection Game – life is an arms race* for effective herbal preparations
Rest: • listen to your symptoms and abide by them • sleep is even more important with illness	I see so many people who push on through acute illness and risk a slow resolution of their disease with all the complications that accompany such. The immune system needs the energy to fight! I find vitamin C to bowel tolerance combined with a good night's sleep has kept me cold free and flu free for 35 years
Heat: • keep warm	Fevers kill all microbes. Some people benefit from sauna-ing. Do not exercise!
Light: • sunshine is best	Sunbathe if possible
Use your brain: • do not suppress symptoms with drugs	Symptoms of infection help the body fight infection. Anti-inflammatory drugs inhibit healing and repair – they allow the microbes to make themselves permanently at home in the body

You may consider that doing all the above amounts to over-kill, but when that next epidemic arrives, as it surely will, you will be very happy to have been prepared and to have these weapons to hand so that you, your family, friends and neighbours will survive. Stock up your Groundhog Acute First Aid box now (see Table A1.3). As Lord Baden Powell wrote in *Scouting for Boys*, 'Be prepared'; and heed the wisdom of Benjamin Franklin (17 January 1706 - 17 April 1790): 'By failing to prepare, you are preparing to fail.'

The contents of the Groundhog Acute Battle First Aid box

John Churchill, 1st Duke of Blenheim (26 May 1650 – 16 June 1722) was a highly successful General, partly because he made sure his armies were fully equipped for battle. The essence of success is to be prepared with the necessary to combat all assailants. As I have said, strike early and strike hard. Of John Churchill, Captain Robert Parker (who was at the Battle of Blenheim, 13 August 1704) wrote: '…it cannot be said that he ever slipped an opportunity of fighting….' We must be equally belligerent in our own individual battles. Part of this belligerence is preparedness, so keep the following in your own 'Battle First Aid Box' and use it at the first sign of attack.

Table A1.3: What to keep in your Battle First Aid box

When	What
For acute infections	
	Vitamin C as ascorbic acid at least 500 g (it is its own preservative so lasts for years) Lugol's iodine 15% – at least 30 ml (it is its own preservative so lasts for years)
Conjunc-tivitis, indeed, any eye infection	Iodine eye drops e.g. Minims povidine iodine 5% OR 2 drops of Lugol's iodine 15% in 5 ml of water; this does not sting the eyes and is the best killer of all microbes in the eye
Upper airway infections	Lugol's iodine – to be used in steam inhalation, OR Salt pipe into which drizzle 4 drops of Lugol's iodine 15% per dose
Skin breaches	Salt – 2 tsp (10 g) in 500 ml water (approx 1 pint) plus 20 ml Lugol's iodine 15%. Use ad lib to wash the wound. Once clean, allow to dry and then smother with iodine oil (coconut oil 100 ml with 10 ml of Lugol's iodine 15% mixed in to make your own ointment or use Providone Iodine Ointment) Plaster or micropore to protect
Fractures	If the skin broken – as for Skin breaches above RICE (rest, ice, elevation – to minimise immediate bleeding and swelling) If the limb is fractured, wrap in cotton wool to protect and bandage abundantly with vet wrap to splint it Next stop… casualty

When	What
Burns	As for skin breaches above. If a large burn, then use cling film to protect once cleaned (put the iodine ointment on the cling film first, then apply to the burn). Protect as per fracture above. For a very large burn… next stop casualty
All injuries involving skin breaches	Sterile dressings: Melolin is a good all-rounder Large roll of cotton wool Crêpe bandages (various sizes) Micropore tape to protect any damaged area from further trauma Vet wrap bandage – this is wonderful stuff, especially if you are in the wilds, to hold it all together
Gastro-enteritis	Sunshine salt: To make up a perfect rehydration drink mix 5 g (1 tsp) in 1 litre of water to give a 0.5% solution
Urine infections	Multistix to test urine D mannose and potassium citrate‡
Bacterial infections	Consider acquiring antibiotics for intelligent use. These should not be necessary if you stick to Groundhog Basic and apply Groundhog Acute. BUT I too live in the real world and am no paragon of virtue, so, if you slip off the band wagon:
Dental	Amoxil 500 mg x 21 capsules
ENT and respiratory	Cephalexin 500 mg three times daily
Diverti-culitis	Doxycycline 100 mg twice daily (DO NOT USE IN PREGNANCY OR FOR CHILDREN)
Urinary	Trimethoprim 200 g twice daily
Any	If you are susceptible to a particular infection, then make sure you always hold the relevant antibiotic; the sooner you treat, the less the damage, but always start with Groundhog Acute

‡Mannose and potassium citrate doses:

D-mannose – One typical product is https://uk.iherb.com/prNow-Foods-D-Mannose-500-mg-120-Veggie-Caps.525. Take 3 x 500 mg capsules one to three times a day

Potassium citrate – These are all example products with their respective doses:

- Effervescent tablets (brand Effercitrate) - take 2 tablets up to three times a day dissolved into a glass of water
- Liquid medicine (brand Cymaclear) - take 2 x 5 ml stirred into a whole glassful of water, up to three times a day
- Sachets (brand Cystopurini) - empty the contents of 1 sachet into a whole glassful of water and stir well before drinking, three times a day.

Putting together such a Battle First Aid Box is as much an intellectual exercise as a practical one and this book, along with our book *The Infection Game – life is an arms race* gives such intellectual imperative. As Shakespeare writes in *Henry V*: 'All things are ready, if our mind be so.'

Groundhog Chronic – what we should all be doing increasingly as we age to live to our full potential

As we age, we acquire infections. My DNA is comprised 15% of retro virus. So is yours. I was inoculated with Salk polio vaccine between 1957 and 1966 so I will probably have simian virus 40, a known carcinogen. I am probably carrying the chickenpox, measles, mumps and rubella viruses because I suffered those as a child. I was also a bit spotty so proprionibacterium acnes may be a potential problem. At least 90% of us have been infected with Epstein Barr virus. I have been bitten by insects and ticks from all over the British Isles so I could also be carrying Lyme (borrelia), bartonella, babesia and perhaps others. I have been a cat owner and could well test positive for bartonella. I have suffered several fractures which have healed but I know within that scar issue will be lurking some microbes – feed them some sugar and they will multiply and give me arthritis. I have had dental abscesses in the past and have one root filling which undoubtably will also harbour microbes. In the past, I have consumed a high carb diet which inevitably results in fermenting gut. On the good side, my puritanical upbringing means I have been free from STDs (thank you Mum!).

All these microbes have the potential to drive nasty diseases such as leukaemia, lymphoma, dementia, Parkinson's, heart disease, auto-immunity, cancer and so on. See *The Infection Game – life is an arms race* for more detail on this. I cannot eliminate them from my body, I have to live with them. I too am part of the Arms Race of the aforementioned book! Of course, this is a race I will (eventually) lose, but I will settle for losing it when I am 100. I am hoping that Groundhog Chronic will handicap my assailants and stack the odds in my favour.

So, as we age and/or we acquire stealth infections, we all need Groundhog Chronic (Table A1.4). It is an extension of Groundhog Basic. Most will end up doing something between the two according to their health and history. But as you get older you have to work harder to stay well.

Table A1.4: Groundhog Chronic

What to do	**Why**	**What I do** My patients always ask me what I do. I am no paragon[§] of virtue, but I may have to become one eventually!
The paleo-ketogenic (PK) diet: • high fat, high fibre, very low carb • probiotic foods like kefir and sauerkraut • no dairy or grains • Two meals a day and no snacking Source the best quality foods you can find and afford – organic is a great start!	See our book *Paleo-Ketogenic – the Why and the How*	Yes. I do the PK diet 95% of the time. 90% organic Glass of cider at weekends! Other liberties if eating out or socialising. But my friends are all becoming PK adapted too
Eat daily food within a 10 hour window of time…	…so 14 hours a day when your stomach is empty – this keeps the stomach acid and so decreases the chances of microbes invading. Maintains ketosis	No breakfast Lunch midday Supper 6.00 pm
Consider episodic fasting one day a week (see our book *Paleo-Ketogenic: The Why and the How)*	This gives the gut a lovely rest and a chance to heal and repair	I do this most weeks. Friday is fast day
A basic package of nutritional supplements – multi-vitamins, multi-minerals and vitamin D 10,000 iu daily	A good multi-vitamin and Sunshine salt 1 tsp daily with food. 1 dsp hemp oil 1 tsp fish oil	Yes

[§]The English noun ‘paragon’ comes from the Italian word *paragone*, which is a touchstone – a black stone that is used to tell the quality of gold.

Table A1.4 *Cont'd*

What to do	**Why**	**What I do** My patients always ask me what I do. I am no paragon[§] of virtue, but I may have to become one eventually!
Glutathione 250 mg daily Iodine 25 mg weekly	We live in such a toxic world we are inevitably exposed. Glutathione and iodine are helpful detox molecules (some people do not tolerate iodine in high doses)	Yes
Vitamin C to 90% of bowel tolerance (most end up on 5 grams). Remember this will change with age, diet and circumstance When you get the dose right you should have no bowel symptoms You can test with urine sticks (page 310) to make sure you have ascorbic acid in your urine – then you have sufficient	With age, influenza becomes a major killer. With Groundhog you need never even get it!	Yes. I currently take 5 grams in the morning. BUT I never get colds or influenza that last more than 24 hours
Lugol's iodine 15% 3 drops daily in water at night	Swill round the mouth and swallow last thing at night. Separate iodine and vitamin C by at least two hours (otherwise they knock each other out – vitamin C is a reducing agent, iodine an oxidising agent)	Yes
Make sure your First Aid box is stocked	So, you have all your ammo to hand to hit new symptoms hard and fast	Yes – even when I go away, I take this – often to treat sickly others!
Sleep 8-9 hours between 10:00 pm and 7:00 am Regular power nap in the day	More in winter, less in summer. Good sleep is as vital as good diet	Yes

What to do	Why	What I do My patients always ask me what I do. I am no paragon[§] of virtue, but I may have to become one eventually!
Exercise within limits. By this I mean you should feel fully recovered next day. If well enough, once a week push those limits, so you get your pulse up to 120 beats per min and all your muscles ache. It is never too late to start! (See Chapter 9)	No pain no gain. Muscle loss is part of ageing - exercise slows this right down Helps to physically dislodge microbes from their hiding places. I suspect massage works similarly	Yes. Thankfully I am one of those who can and who enjoys exercise I garden, walk and ride plus 20 press-ups and 20 squats every morning
Take supplements for the raw materials for connective tissue such as glucosamine. Bone broth is the best!	With age we become less good at healing and repair	Yes
Herbs, spices and fungi in cooking	Use your favourite herbs, spices and fungi in cooking and food, and lots of them!	Yes. Because I love food!
Consider herbs to improve the defences	Astragalus, cordyceps and rhodiola can easily be incorported into your PK diet	Sometimes when in stock and I remember
Address energy delivery mechanisms as below	See this book!	Yes, Craig– I've got the book![¶]
Take the mitochondrial package of supplements daily vis: CoQ10 100 g, niacinamide slow release 1500 mg, acetyl L carnitine 500 mg. D ribose 5-10 grams at night if you have really overdone things	With age fatigue becomes an increasing issue because our mitochondrial engines start to slow. The ageing process is determined by mitochondria. Look after them!	Yes I don't take carnitine because I eat meat and my digestion is good

[¶]Sarah has commented thus: 'Yes, Craig – I've got the book!' This is a reference to our consultations. Often Sarah is heard to say (in answer to my many questions): 'It's in that book, the one you wrote,' to which I answer: 'Yes, Sarah – I've got the book!'

Table A1.4 *Cont'd*

What to do	**Why**	**What I do** My patients always ask me what I do. I am no paragon[§] of virtue, but I may have to become one eventually!
Mitochondria may be going slow because of toxins. Consider tests of toxic load to see if you need to do any detox	A good all-rounder is Genova urine screen with DMSA 15 mg per kg of body weight. You can get this test through https://smartnutrition.co.uk/health-tests/toxic-heavy-metals/	This is the only test I have ever done on myself! It showed background levels of toxic minerals
	Most other toxins can be eliminated with heating regimes and shower off after (see Chapter 14)	My favourite is an Epsom Salts bath
Check your living space for electromagnetic pollution	You can buy good EMF detectors relatively cheaply (£30), for example, ERICKHILL EMF detectors are good and well priced	Yes. The cordless phone has gone! I never hold a mobile phone to my ear – I use the speaker. Turn wifi off at night – have now moved to ethernet
Review any prescription medication – they are all potential toxins! The need for drugs is likely to be symptomatic of failure to apply Groundhog	Ask yourself why you are taking drugs? See our book *Ecological Medicine*. Once Groundhog is in place many drugs can be stopped. Taking prescription drugs is the third commonest cause of death in Westerners	I never take symptom-suppressing medication. This has allowed full and now pain-free recovery from three broken necks (horses again) and other fractures
Consider tests of adrenal and thyroid function since these glands fatigue with age and chronic infection	Thyroid bloods tests and adrenal saliva tests are available through labs as listed in Useful resources (page 303) and see our book *The Underactive Thyroid: Do it yourself because your doctor won't*	I find glandulars very helpful and currently take thyroid glandular 60 mg in the morning and 60 mg midday. Pregnenolone 50 mg once daily

What to do	Why	What I do My patients always ask me what I do. I am no paragon§ of virtue, but I may have to become one eventually!
Heat and light	Always keep warm. Sunbathe at every opportunity. Holidays in warm climates with sunbathing and swimming are excellent for killing infections and detoxing Do not forget hyperthermia and light are a good treatment for chronic infections	I am a pyromaniac! My kitchen is lovely and warm with a wood-fired range. I work in my conservatory with natural light. I sunbathe as often as wet Wales permits.
Use your brain	Foresight: Avoid risky actions like kissing†, unprotected sex Caution: Avoid vaccinations. Choose travel destinations with care. Circumspection: Do not symptom suppress with drugs, treat breaches of the skin seriously	I have to say that with age this is much less of an issue! No vaccinations. No foreign travel to countries where vaccines are needed

If you are tiring from Groundhog, be inspired by these quotations:

We are what we repeatedly do. Excellence, then, is not an act, but a habit.

Idiomatic translation by Will Durrant in *The Story of Philosophy*' of the original

Excellence is an art won by training and habituation…

Aristotle, 384 – 322 BCE

repetitio est mater studiorum – repetition is the mother of all learning.

Old Latin Proverb

consuetudinis magna vis est – the force of habit is great.

Cicero, 106 – 43 BCE

Assassinated for his opposition to Mark Antony, Cicero's last words were purportedly:

There is nothing proper about what you are doing, soldier, but do try to kill me properly.

Appendix 2

Diet, detox and die-off (DDD) reactions

- Expect to get worse
- See this as a good sign
- Why this happens
- What to do about it.

'The darkest hour is before dawn'

Old English Proverb now universally used*

Expect to get worse before you improve. The sickest patients get the worst reactions, so the regimes have to be put in place slowly. This may be demoralising but it depends how you see it… and I am an optimist so I see progress in the right direction. Such reactions are a well-recognised phenomenon and are given comforting names such as a 'healing crisis'. Symptoms can be very severe. Often when patients are so ill, they cannot afford to become any worse. I have great sympathy but no easy answers. Understanding the

*__Footnote:__ The English theologian and historian, Thomas Fuller (19 June 1608 – 16 August 1661), is perhaps the first person to commit this phrase to the printed word. His religious travelogue, *A Pisgah-Sight Of Palestine And The Confines Thereof*, 1650, contains this sentence: 'It is always darkest just before the Day dawneth.' Meant metaphorically, this phrase is not 'actually' true although it can be said that it is coldest before dawn. (Please see https://davidson.weizmann.ac.il/en/online/askexpert/sky-darkest-just-dawn for more detail on this[1]) Sometimes, just before sunrise, the sun casts a shadow of the earth into the visible sky and this gives an impression of a sweep of darkness, much akin to that experienced in a total solar eclipse. It could be that this sweep of darkness gave a 'physical' truth to this phrase and led to its common use.

mechanisms may help. You must be a patient patient.

Also expect a bumpy ride – die-off reactions do not follow a smooth course. Be prepared for something like this:

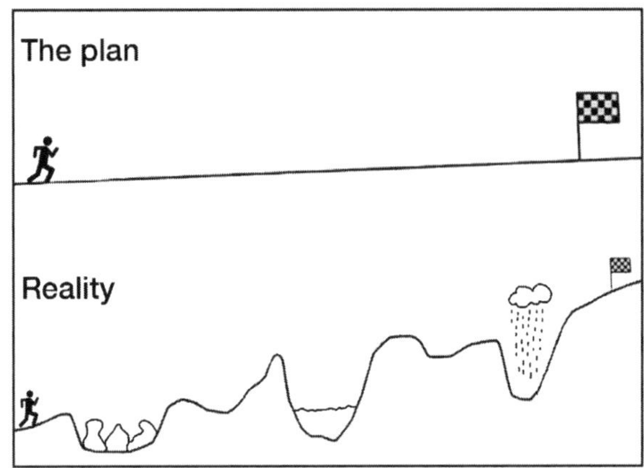

We are fighting a war, but this is composed of many battles. Battles are fought by the macrophage foot soldiers and the lymphocyte officers of our immune system. They can be activated by infections, allergies, autoimmunity and toxins. The army throws its all at the invaders and kills them with cytokine bullets. The inflammatory friendly fire that results makes us feel ill. Then the immune armies rest and recover (we feel a bit better) before attacking again – I told you it was a bumpy ride! Then the immune system sweeps up the mess – the parts of dead microbes look like the parts of live ones and this explains 'Herx' reactions (see below).

Diet reactions – there are three common players

1. The metabolic hinterland

The transition from burning carbs to burning fat is difficult and takes time – usually one or two weeks. The body has been used to running on carbs and there is an inertia in the system – it is as if it takes time to 'learn' to burn fat. During this window of time the body cannot get fuel from carbs (because they have been cut out of the diet) so it uses adrenalin to burn fat. To the patient this gives some of the symptoms of low blood sugar because adrenalin is partly responsible for such. We call this 'keto flu', but it is also given the dreadful and confusing name of 'ketogenic hypoglycaemia'. It was first described in the 1960s in children treated for epilepsy with a ketogenic diet. Let me explain further.

We experience the collective symptoms of low blood sugar not only for reasons of low blood sugar, but also for the hormonal response to such:

- Poor energy delivery due to low blood sugar: fatigue, foggy brain and (indeed for some, especially diabetics on medication) loss of consciousness
- Adrenalin release: feeling 'hyper', shaky, anxious, possibly with palpitations and fast heart rate
- Gut hormones: feelings of hunger and the need to eat.

If all is well with the metabolism, the body switches into fat-burning mode (as I've said, it takes one to two weeks for this to happen) and all the above symptoms, which we associate with low blood sugar, disappear. If all is not well with the metabolism, then these symptoms do not disappear and the clinical picture which results is called 'ketogenic hypoglycaemia'. I suspect two causes: lack of carnitine (easily corrected with 1 gram daily) and, more commonly, lack of sufficient thyroid hormone to burn fat. That clinical picture is characterised by:

- normal or (even better) low and stable blood sugar levels
- ketosis (confirmed by blood and urine tests)
- the body is burning fat to produce ketones, but it does not have sufficient thyroid hormone to do so efficiently – it relies on extra adrenalin to burn fat
- BUT the adrenalin release gives us nasty symptoms of being 'hyper', shaky, anxious, possibly with palpitations and fast heart rate
- AND gut hormone release – which 'follow' adrenalin release – that is, feelings of hunger and the need to eat
- Clinically, this feels like hypoglycaemia.

Analyse your symptoms. We know keto-adapted athletes improve their performance and the foggy brain clears… despite perhaps feeling dreadful in other respects.

To treat ketogenic hypoglycaemia I recommend: acetyl L carnitine 2 grams daily, and sort out the thyroid problem. But we have to go gently here. In the short term, thyroid and adrenal hormones have very similar actions – that is, to speed things up. If one is still in the metabolic hinterland you may still be spiking adrenalin as your body has yet to 'learn' to use thyroid to burn fat. If you add thyroid hormones to this mix you will end up with the combined effects of thyroid hormones and adrenalin and feel constantly 'hyper'. (See our book *The Underactive Thyroid* for how to manage this.)

2. Addiction reactions

We use addiction to mask unpleasant symptoms such as fatigue, foggy brain and/or pain. Stop the addiction and those symptoms return – ghastly in the short term, great in the long. Obviously sugar and starch addiction are illustrated by the metabolic hinterland[†] but chocolate, caffeine, alcohol, nicotine, cola and other such all have the potential to cause 'train spotting' pain.

3. Allergy reactions

Allergy and addiction seem to be two sides of the same coin. I once had a patient who, even before I was allowed to introduce myself, declared that when he died, he would like to take a cow to heaven with him to ensure a supply of his favourite food. The diagnosis was not difficult. I am not sure of the mechanism by which allergy has this addictive effect, but it is very real.

Detoxification reactions

In the short term, the body can deal with a spike of some toxins by stuffing these into fat and thereby out of harm's way. When I do fat biopsies, results come back in milligrams per kilogram. By contrast, blood results come back in micrograms per kilogram. This alone tells us toxic levels in fat are a thousand-fold higher than in blood. Losing weight, heating fat or perhaps even physical massage mobilises these toxins into the bloodstream

[†]**Independent film note by Craig**: One of my favourite films is *Hinterland* (not to be confused with the BBC series of the same name). This film is an independent British feature, written and directed by Harry Macqueen. You can sometimes find it here: www.amazon.co.uk/Hinterland-Harry-Macqueen/dp/B00VA61A34. It is the story of an old friendship rekindled, and of self-discovery and heartbreak. Yes, I know – I am such a soppy git! Craig

and cause an acute poisoning. These toxins, especially pesticides and volatile organic compounds (VOCs), 'boil off' through the skin with heating regimes and cause rashes as the skin reacts allergically to them passing through. The commonest include urticaria and acne-like rashes. The clue can be found in the skin reaction to organochlorine poisoning, so called 'chloracne'. I have seen several patients who have been chemically poisoned develop acne whilst detoxing with heat treatments (such as sauna-ing), persist with treatment regardless and eventually find their acne reaction resolved. I can explain this only by a reaction to toxins as they are excreted through the skin.

Some patients being treated with vitamin B12 by injection and/or iodine also get an acne reaction. Both B12 and iodine are good at mobilising toxins from the body. Again, this resolves with time if the sufferer is prepared to put up with the acne in the short term.

Heavy metals stick to proteins and bioconcentrate in organs, particularly the brain, heart, kidneys and bone. They can be mobilised nutritional and chelation, and this too may result in detox reactions.

Mobilising such chemicals is akin to throwing a handful of sand into a finely tuned engine; this may produce almost any symptom. In the very short term, energy delivery mechanism will be impaired. Many toxic metals and chemicals are immuno-toxic – that is, they switch on inflammation.

Die-off reactions ('Herx' or 'Herxheimer')

Die-off reactions were first described by two immunologists, Drs Jarisch and Herxheimer, in patients with syphilis treated with antimicrobials. These symptoms are partly due to endotoxin-like products released by the death of micro-organisms within the body and partly by immune activation. (I think of this as 'allergy to dead microbes', which may explain why Herx reactions are not universal.) Such reactions are potentially very serious and must always be taken as such by at least reducing the dose of any antimicrobial employed and relaxing the regimes that may have triggered the reactions. In the treatment of chronic infection with antimicrobials, I suggest starting with a tiny dose and building up slowly over a few days. The sicker the patient, the more likely they are to get a 'Herx'.

Symptoms of diet, detox and die-off

In practice I have found one can experience:

- Inflammation:
    - systemic symptoms (fever, malaise, aches and pains, depression and fatigue) or local symptoms (acute cold, cough, catarrh, diarrhoea, cystitis etc). See Chapter 10 for symptoms of inflammation.
    - local symptoms: it seems to be characteristic of sniffing with an iodine salt pipe that there is an initial increase in mucus and catarrh production; I suspect that as the iodine kills the microbes the body recognises them as invaders and sweeps them out with snot.
    - It is important stuff. As consultant immunologist and dear friend, Dr David Freed, used to say: 'It may be snot to you but it's my bread and butter.'
- Fatigue: when the immune system is active it takes all our energy, so there is none available to spend physically.
- Foggy brain: the inflamed body is paralleled by the inflamed brain and symptoms of poor energy delivery to the brain result, in particular, with foggy brain, depression and malaise.
- Sickness behaviour: 'Leave me alone. I just wanna go to bed!' This is an energy-saving strategy.

Table A2.1: Summary: Getting worse with Groundhog regimes when they should be making you better

Problem	**Mechanisms**	**Action**
Metabolic hinterland with ketogenic hypoglycaemia...	Adrenalin is high	Stick with the PK diet. Measure ketones to make sure you are in ketosis. See Useful resources (page 303) for ketone measuring devices. Allow two weeks
...if this persists	Hypothyroidism	Sort out your thyroid with our book *The Underactive Thyroid*. T3 is the fat burner
	Lack of carnitine	You need acetyl L carnitine to burn fat. I suggest 2 grams daily for two months, then a maintenance dose of 500 mg daily (but with a good PK diet, this should not be necessary in the long term)

Problem	Mechanisms	Action
	'Glycogen storage disorder'[‡] (GSD)	This may be associated with poor adrenal function – work out the cause
Detox reactions	Acute poisoning as chemicals are mobilised from fat	Heating regimes bring toxins out through the skin and this reduces the poisoning effect. Consider zeolite clays which adsorb (not absorb) fat soluble toxins in bile to pull them out in faeces
Addiction withdrawal symptoms in response to withdrawal of social, recreational (this really is a misnomer) and/or prescription drugs	Addiction masks unpleasant symptoms	If too awful then take a tiny dose of your addiction and wean yourself off slowly. I dreaded the prospect of giving up caffeine, but when I made up my mind it was easy[§]
Allergen withdrawal, typically grains or dairy	Do not know for sure – many possibilities	Stick with the PK diet If you really get stuck do a carnivore diet (see our book *Paleo-Ketogenic: The Why and the How* and also Chapter 4 of this book)
Symptoms as micronutrient status improves	Mobilising and excreting toxic metals	Consider clays (I use diatomaceous earth or 'food clays' which adsorb fat-soluble metals in bile to pull them out in faeces) then take a tiny dose of your addiction and wean yourself off slowly.
Symptoms from heating regimes and/or weight loss	Mobilising pesticides and VOCs from fat	Difficult – slow the regimes down to a point that is bearable

[‡]**Footnote:** GSD is a metabolic disorder caused by enzyme deficiencies. It can affect glycogen synthesis, glycogen breakdown or glycolysis – glucose breakdown – and it typically occurs with muscle and/or liver cells. It can be genetic or acquired.

[§]**Footnote on caffeine from Craig:** Sarah is not alone in her love of caffeine. I drink green tea every day and I make a cup of coffee for my wife, Penny, first thing in the morning every day too. It is on record that 89% of Americans consume some caffeine every day of their lives.[2] According to new research, humans have been drinking beverages containing caffeine since at least 750 AD.[3]

Table A2.1 *Cont'd*

Problem	Mechanisms	Action
Symptoms from reducing microbial loads with Groundhog Acute or antimicrobial drugs	Herx reactions	Relax the regime and then once tolerated, get up to speed again
Adrenalin spiking with high blood sugar, blood pressure and/or loss of sleep	Any one of the above is a stress and the body responds with adrenalin	Stick with it and hang on to your hat!¶
Skin rashes: urticaria, itching, acne	'Allergic' reactions to toxins coming through the skin	Stick with it! It will pass and as it does so other symptoms will improve

All the above illustrates the point that time is a vital part of the diagnostic and therapeutic process. I expect patients to get to this stage after an initial consultation with me that usually concludes with me saying, 'You may love me now, but in a week's time you will hate me'. It is no consolation to tell them that I too have been on the same journey and been equally grumpy about the whole proces. I am sure Craig has experienced the same. (Craig: Indeed, I have but I have never 'hated' Sarah! When going through these DDD reactions, I always have Penny on hand to remind me, 'This is just what Sarah said might happen!')

¶**Footnote:**: This expression may derive from the need to do just this on rollercoaster rides, according to lexicographer Eric Partridge (Colloquial; first half of 1900s). This rather suits the 'Reality' graphic on page 248. Eric Honeywood Partridge (6 February 1894 – 1 June 1979) was a New Zealand–British lexicographer of the English language, particularly of its slang.

Appendix 3

Commonly used blood tests and what they mean

Poor interpretations have led to some serious mistakes throughout history. Even St Jerome, the patron saint of translators, fell victim: he translated the Old Bible from Hebrew and made a simple error concerning the moment when Moses came down from Mount Sinai, with his head in 'radiance'. In Hebrew, *karan* means radiance, but because Hebrew is written without vowels, St Jerome read '*karan*'as '*keren*', which means 'horned'. Because of this mistake there are many paintings and sculptures of Moses with horns. More recently, in 1980 Willie Ramírez was admitted to a Florida hospital in a comatose state. At the time of admission, an interpreter translated the Spanish term '*intoxicado*',which means 'poisoned' or having had an allergic reaction, as 'intoxicated'. Willie, who was suffering from an intracerebral haemorrhage, was treated for an intentional drug overdose. As a result, he was left quadriplegic. This resulted in a $71million malpractice suit. Other examples of poor interpretation include those listed in Table A3.1.

Table A3.1: Significant mis-translations

Speaker	What they said/intended	How it was interpreted
US President Jimmy Carter speaking to a Polish audience	'...I have come to learn your opinions and understand your desires for the future...'	'I desire the Poles carnally...'
HSBC marketing campaign	'Assume nothing...'	'Do nothing...'

Table A3.1 *Cont'd*

Speaker	What they said/intended	How it was interpreted
Japanese Prime Minister Kantaro Suzuki, referring to the Potsdam conference in 1945*	'No comment. We are still thinking about it'	'We are ignoring it in contempt.'
On 6 August 1945, four days after this comment was mis-translated, the American bomber 'Enola Gay' dropped a five-ton atomic bomb over the Japanese city of Hiroshima		
During US President Richard Nixon's visit to China in 1972, Chinese premier Zhou Enlai famously said it was 'too early to tell' when evaluating the effects of the French Revolution	Zhou Enlai was referring to the 1968 riots in Paris	The comments were interpreted as referring to the French Revolution in 1789 and the Western press inferred great wisdom in the Chinese Premier's words and compared how the East always took the long view as opposed to the shabby short-term West
Italian astronomer Giovanni Virginio Schiaparelli mapped Mars in 1877, calling dark and light areas on the planet's surface as 'seas' and 'continents' and labelling what he thought were channels with the Italian word 'canali'	Virginio was trying to describe what he saw in everyday language	Canali was mis-translated as 'canals' and there followed a belief that 'life on Mars' had been established. Even respected figures such as US astronomer Percival Lowell mapped hundreds of these 'canals' between 1894 and 1895 and published three books on Mars with illustrations showing what he thought were artificial structures built to carry water by a brilliant race of engineers

Having said that, this Appendix really should not be necessary. But I daily see medical tests that have been poorly interpreted so vital clues are missed. This is for several reasons:

[*]**Historical note:** The heads of Government of the UK, USA and USSR held this conference to consider the post-WWII order, the formal peace treaty and countering the effects of the war… as these three issues concerned the defeated Germany. The conference ended 2 August 1945.

- If a test result lies within the reference ranges, then the patient is told it is normal and that no action is required. However, while reference ranges reflect population averages, some individuals will function best at the top end of the range, and some others at the low end of the range.
- Population ranges may not reflect normal ranges. Ranges are arrived at by measuring the current population, which may not be normal. The best example is levels of T4 (thyroxine) in the blood – the reference range for the lab I use is 12-22 pmol/l, but some NHS labs have ranges as low as 7-14 pmol/l. This will result in missing many cases of secondary hypothyroidism. Population ranges are not normal ranges.
- Ranges have changed even in my lifetime. A normal blood sugar level used to be 4-6.8 mmol/l, but now levels up to 11 mmol/l are considered acceptable by some.
- A range may be negatively skewed[†]. A normal range for a white cell count is often 4-11, but most people run normally at 4-6. A white cell count running consistently above this (above 6) may point to chronic inflammation.

The key point is that tests are there to narrow the diagnosis, not to make it. All diagnosis is hypothesis which then depends on response to treatment. All diagnosis is therefore retrospective!

Table A3.2 covers commonly performed tests which I often see badly interpreted. It is not exhaustive.

[†]**Negative skew:** A distribution is 'skewed' if one of its tails is longer than the other. The distribution in Figure A3.1 has a negative skew since it has a long tail in the negative (left) direction.

Figure A3.1: Histogram of age at death of Australian males in 2012

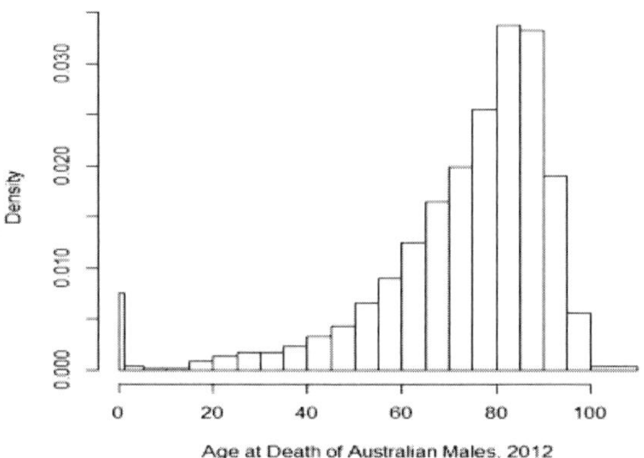

Table A3.2: Commonly misinterpreted test results

Test	Significant result	What it means	Action
Full blood count	Haemoglobin: Men 140-160 g/l Women 130-145 g/l	If low (anaemia), reasons could be: not making blood fast enough because of deficiency in a raw material or lacking the energy for manufacture	Do faecal occult blood test to check for losses from the gut… and for faecal calprotectin, both of which may indicate pathology Check if heavy periods are an issue Ferritin test to check for iron deficiency Measure homocysteine – see below
		If too high, reasons could be: smoker? polycythaemia rubra vera carbon monoxide poisoning	Stop smoking and recheck See a doctor
	MCV (mean corpuscular volume) 87-94 fl	If too high, reasons could be: hypothyroid poor methylator postal delay between blood taking and blood testing may cause a false macrocytosis (enlargement of red blood cells)	See Chapter 7 and/or read our book *The Underactive Thyroid* Measure homocysteine. It is possible your GP can do this test. High homocysteine is a risk factor for fatigue but also arterial disease, cancer and dementia, so this is an important test, not least because if positive then you must screen all first-degree relatives as high homocysteine runs in families. Alternatively, DIY test with www.cerascreen.co.uk/products/homocysteine-test Check time between sample taking and testing
		If low, reasons could be iron deficiency thalassaemia or a haemoglobin variant heavy metal poisoning	Check ferritin Blood test for haemoglobinopathy Urine test for heavy metals with DMSA (see page 141)

Test	Significant result	What it means	Action
	WCC (white cell count) – the normal range is positively skewed, so I expect to see a result of 4-6 (x 10 to the power of 9/l)	If high: this may be a short-term response to acute infection If constantly high	Repeat in two weeks Consult a doctor (cancers may present with high WCC) Look for cause of inflammation
		If low: white cells being used up fast to fight infection AND/OR lack of raw materials AND/OR lack of energy to make white cells	Improve energy delivery mechanisms Improve nutritional status Identify the infection (see our book *The Infection Game*) – the commonest offenders in ME are EBV, Lyme and mycoplasma
	Platelets should be 150-350 (x 10 to the power of 9/l)	Too high: may point to B12 deficiency	Measure active B12 and homocysteine
		Too low: may point to autoimmunity	See doctor to consider Idiopathic thrombocytopenic purpura (ITP)
		If below 100 see doctor urgently	
		Below 100 may mean poor bone marrow function	Check quality and quantity of red cells and white cells – if all low then this is bone marrow suppression which could be due to exhaustion of chronic infection, poisoning, poor energy delivery mechanisms

Table A3.2 *Cont'd*

Test	Significant result	What it means	Action
	ESR <5 mm/ hour C reactive protein <1.0 nmol/l Plasma viscosity 1.5-1.65 mPA	These are all measures of inflammation. Reference ranges have all been increased because so many people are inflamed as a result of metabolic syndrome. An ESR up to 20 is now considered acceptable!	If inflammatory markers are raised, always ask the question 'why?' I suspect a high ESR is due to poor quality fourth phase water (see page 155) – this makes for sticky blood (see DMSO, Chapter 16)
Choles-terol	Total cholesterol – reference ranges are set too low – I like to see 6-8 mmol/l	If high, may be due to: hypothyroidism vitamin D deficiency If too low, you starve the brain and immune system of this essential fat	See Chapter 7 re underactive thyroid Measure vitamin D (I like to see this 175-250 nmol/l) Eat PK (Chapter 4) and get plenty of sunshine
		A British study in 1995 found those with a cholesterol level below 4.8 mmol/l had the highest all-cause mortality[1]. 19 studies have linked raised cholesterol with longevity in the elderly.[2] The Honolulu Heart Program followed 3572 elderly Japanese/American men for 20 years and found those with low cholesterol on two occasions measured 20 years apart had the highest mortality[3]	Eat a high-fat diet – of course the PK diet (Chapter 2) is high-fat, high-fibre
	LDL cholesterol 2-4.4 mmol/l	A high LDL is not dangerous – LDL is not 'bad' cholesterol Cholesterol is carried in the blood as cholesterol sulphate. High LDL may point to low sulphate	Glutathione 250 mg daily Epsom salt baths DMSO 20 ml daily – all help to replenish sulphate (and much more too)

Test	Significant result	What it means	Action
	HDL cholesterol <2.0 mmol/l	Suggests HDL is being used up in the business of healing and repairing arteries – i.e. they are being damaged by something. This may be metabolic syndrome and/ or high uric acid and/or high homocysteine and/or chronic inflammation	PK diet Check uric acid and homocysteine Look for inflammation
	HDL cholesterol >2.0 mmol/l	The percentage of 'friendly' HDL is good. HDL is *not* being used up in the business of healing and repairing arteries – i.e. they are in good shape	
	Triglycerides high >1.0 mmol/l	To test accurately, this *must* be an overnight fasting sample and should be <1.0 mmol/l	Triglycerides may be raised if you have recently consumed medium-chain fats (which is fine) OR because you have high insulin and high blood sugar, so insulin is shunting sugar into triglycerides (not fine)
Electrolytes	Sodium (Na): I like to see 140–144 mmol/l	If low either there is: a lack of salt in the diet or a salt-losing state e.g. diuretics or kidney failure	On a PK diet the need for salt increases – aim for 5 grams daily (1 teaspoonful of Sunshine Salt)
		If <135 mmol/l…	…you need to see a doctor as a matter of urgency
	Potassium (K[‡]): I like to see 4.0-4.4 mmol/l	If high, there may have been a delay in transport – K easily leaks out of cells	Check the time between sample taking and testing If above 4.9 mmol/l you need to see a doctor as a matter of urgency

[‡]**Linguistic note**: Why is the symbol for potassium 'K'? 'Potassium' is derived from the English word potash. The chemical symbol 'K' comes from 'kalium', the Mediaeval Latin for potash, which may have derived from the Arabic word *qali*, meaning alkali. Interested readers should see https://en.wikipedia.org/wiki/ Symbol_(chemistry)

Table A3.2 *Cont'd*

Test	Significant result	What it means	Action
		If low, it may be because: too little in the diet diuretics waste potassium	The body cannot store potassium – you have to eat it daily. There is plenty in the PK diet Take Sunshine Salt If <3.5 mmol/l then see a doctor urgently
	Corrected calcium (Ca) 2.35-2.55 mmol/l	If low: this points to vitamin D deficiency	Measure vitamin D
		If high: this must always be taken seriously!	Consult a doctor urgently if above 2.8 mmol/l – you may have hyperparathyroidism
	Serum magnesium (Mg) 0.8-0.95 mmol/l	Rarely done as this is not a reliable test of body stores. Most doctors do not understand the difference between a serum Mg and a red cell Mg. Serum levels must be kept within a tight range, or the heart stops. Therefore, serum levels are maintained at the expense of levels inside cells	Ignore if normal If <0.7 mmol/l then you are in serious trouble and need urgent medical attention
	Creatinine 60-110 mcmol/l	Too high suggests: a high protein diet and/or high muscle mass or poor kidney function	Reduce protein intake and recheck Look for causes of kidney damage
		Too low points to: low protein diet and/or low muscle mass Smaller people and women have less muscle mass so interpret this in that light	Eat more protein Take more exercise Smaller people and women may be perfectly fit but carry a smaller muscle mass

Test	Significant result	What it means	Action
	Urea <7.0 mmol/l	If high this suggests dehydration	You need water *and* fat *and* salt *and* sulphate to be properly hydrated
		High urea may accompany high creatinine	See creatinine above
	Uric acid high if >300 mcmol/l (or 5 mg/dl)	Uric acid is a mycotoxin 80% comes from fructose and sucrose 20% comes from protein	Look for a fungal issue – see Chapter 20 Cut out fructose – the main source is fruit sugar including corn syrup
	12 hour fasting glucose 4.0-5.6 fl (ideally lower than 5.0)	If higher then you are on the way to diabetes If you are keto-adapted, then low blood sugar presents no problem at all	PK diet
	Glycosylated haemoglobin 22-38 mmol/mol 39-46 is prediabetes Above 46 is diabetes	A very useful test of average blood sugar over the past three months. Ranges have changed recently because nearly all Westerners eat too much carb and are on the way to diabetes. How can the NHS deal with this? Move the goal posts	PK diet See our books *Prevent & Cure Diabetes* and *Paleo-Ketogenic: The Why and the How*
		The lower the better. On a good PK diet this may be less than 30. I would settle for less than 34	

Table A3.2 *Cont'd*

Test	**Significant result**	**What it means**	**Action**
Liver function tests	GGT (gamma-glutamyl transpeptidase) below 20 IU/l ALT (alanine transaminase) below 20 IU/l AST (aspartate amino-transferase) below 20 IU/l	Standard reference ranges are all set higher than those listed here because so many people are poisoned If raised, then this is due to enzyme induction to deal with toxins. This is not liver damage. However, if the alkaline phosphatase is also high then you are progressing to liver damage The commonest toxins are …..	The commonest toxins are: • Alcohol typically increases gamma GT • Other drugs may also cause enzyme induction • Consider toxins from the outside world - see Chapter 14 • Consider products of the upper fermenting gut (page 40) • Monitor alkaline phosphatase for liver damage
	Alkaline phosphatase high Should be <80 IU/l	I like to see this below 80, *otherwise* it suggests mild liver damage. Note the liver is very good at healing and repairing itself	Find the cause! The commonest cause is a carbohydrate-based diet
	LDH (lactate dehydrogenase) 150-200 U/l	There may be any tissue damage in the body commonly of liver, bones, heart, kidneys	What is the cause of tissue damage? Consult a doctor
		I suspect where there are poor energy delivery mechanisms with early switch into anaerobic metabolism inducing this enzyme	Improve energy delivery mechanisms
	Bilirubin <12 mcmol/l	If high, this means you are a slow detoxifier via glucuronidation and will be more susceptible to toxic stress. When it is above 19 this is called Gilbert's syndrome	Identify the cause of the toxic stress and mitigate - see Chapter 14. Take glutathione 250 mg for life to improve liver detox

Test	Significant result	What it means	Action
Bone		Having normal 'bone markers' does not exclude osteoporosis	The best test for osteoporosis is a heel bone density scan with ultrasound. This is accurate and involves no ionising radiation
	Phosphate 0.97-1.20 mmol/l	If high	Check for kidney disease (see doctor)
		If low, points to vitamin D deficiency	Measure vitamin D Check for kidney disease and parathormone levels (see doctor)
	Ferritin: Men 30-300 ng/ml Women 30-150 ng/ml	If low, you are iron deficient because of: losing blood from the gut losing blood from heavy periods Low iron intake due to • insufficient iron in diet • malabsorption (upper fermenting gut?)	Check faecal occult blood and faecal calprotectin Check gynae history Increase iron (meat) in the diet PK diet
		If high: points to inflammation	Look for causes of inflammation.
		If very high: may point to haemochromatosis	See a doctor and get gene tested
Prostate	PSA <2.0 ng/ml	PSA reflects the amount of prostate tissue. Western diets high in carbs and dairy stimulate growth. This means reference ranges have been changed so older men have a higher range	Regardless of the result, do the PK diet
		If high, remember it is the rate of change that suggests malignancy, not the absolute amount.	Keep rechecking monthly and arrange for MRI scan of the prostate gland Go PK – this may shrink the prostate gland and reduce the PSA

Table A3.2 *Cont'd*

Test	Significant result	What it means	Action
B12	Total B12 200-900 ng/ml I like to see >2000 ng/ml	'Normal' ranges simply reflect that which prevents pernicious anaemia, not what will support optimal biochemical function. NB: Much of the total B12 is inactive	A 'normal' B12 never predicts a response to B12 by injection Neither does it accurately predict the level of active B12
	A better measure is active B12 (HoloTC) >50 pg/ml		To be sure, also measure homocysteine
Homo-cysteine	I like to see this between 5 and 10 mcmol/l (NB: Many lab reference ranges state <15 mcmol/l	High (or low) homocysteine tells us you are a poor methylator and/or do not have the raw materials. Methylation is an essential biochemical tool to allow one to 'read' DNA, to detoxify, to synthesise enzymes and proteins and much more. Being a poor methylator is a *major* risk factor for arterial disease, dementia, cancer and degenerative disease. And of course CFS	To correct this you need to take methylated B vitamins: • pyridoxal 5 phosphate 50 mg (in most good multivitamins) • methyl folic acid (MTHFA) 800 mcg • methylated B12 5 mg • glutathione 250 mg daily for life. This usually does the trick but some need methyl B12 by injection Must retest after four months of the above Whatever regime works, continue it for life and check episodically to make sure the regimes are effective
		This a genetic lesion	At the least, first-degree relatives should be screened, or any relative with a poor family history of arterial disease, cancer or dementia

Test	Significant result	What it means	Action
Thyroid	TSH <1.5 mIU/l	Low or normal TSH never excludes the possibility of secondary hypothyroidism due to poor pituitary function NB: A TSH tells us little but it is relied upon far too heavily by many doctors to determine the dose of thyroid hormone	Also see our book *The Underactive Thyroid*
	Free T4 12-22 pmol/l	Check the reference range. Some NHS ranges are as low as 7-14 pmol/l	Be aware that some people do not feel well until running at 30 pmol/l
	Free T3 3.1-6.8 pmol/l	Ditto above	Ditto above
		If T3 is low compared to T4: this suggests poor conversion of inactive T4 to the active T3 – i.e. T3 hypothyroidism	You may need a T3 supplement
		If TSH is high despite good levels of T4 and T3: this points to thyroid hormone receptor resistance	Consider measuring reverse T3 level Look for a toxic cause
	High reverse T3 0.13-0.35 nmol/l	If high: This points to thyroid hormone receptor resistance, in which event blood tests are not helpful	You must rely on the clinical picture to determine the dose of thyroid hormone - again see out book *The Underactve Thyroid*
Vitamin D	At least 125 nmol/l Ideally nearer 200	A recent study showed that having a vitamin D level above 125 nmol/l (50 ng/ml) affords a risk of death from covid-19 that is effectively zero[4]	We all need 10,000 iu daily. If you are off all dairy and not taking calcium supplements then it is safe to take 20,000 iu daily. The only possible toxicity of vitamin D is high calcium

Test	Significant result	What it means	Action
		The anti-inflammatory effects of vitamin D really cut in at 160 nmol/l or higher	
Adrenal stress test (saliva)	High levels of cortisol	This indicates a chronic stress response. The commonest cause of this is a hypoglycaemic tendency of metabolic syndrome (this is a pre-diabetic condition). The problem is also that this is not sustainable in the long term – eventually the adrenal gland will fatigue. Other causes of stress may be work, financial, physical, emotional etc	Work out the cause of the stress
		DHEA low and/or not commensurate with the cortisol response. This is typical of early adrenal fatigue	See our book *The Underactive Thyroid* Pregnenolone 5 mg sublingually on rising is a good start
	Flat cortisol with no waking spike	Underactive thyroid	See our book *The Underactive Thyroid*

Appendix 4

State welfare benefits – UK

UK Government Spring Budget 2023

The UK Government launched a Health and Disability White Paper in its Spring Budget 2023.[1] A key plank is to remove the Work Capability Assessment (WCA) so that in future there will be only one health and disability assessment – the Personal Independent Payment (PIP) assessment. The idea is that for Universal Credit claimants, the WCA will be removed and replaced with a new Universal Credit health element. So, this should reduce the number of health assessments that people claiming both PIP and UC will need to take to access their benefits.

The new system will be rolled out, to new claims only, on a staged, geographical basis from no earlier than 2026/27. The new claims roll-out is expected be completed within three years, by 2029 at the earliest. The discussion that follows in this section refers to the existing WCA, and, as you can see from the expected roll-out timetable, the WCA will still be the main method of assessment for many years to come.

Introduction

It is beyond the scope of this book to give a detailed account of all the benefits that may be available in individual circumstances, but it is an important area where I can give some guidance based on my experiences of these matters and also where I can signpost to further sources of support and information.

For a list of patient-generated sources of support go to the following link; not all of these relate to welfare benefits but see Section 4 which covers this: www.drmyhill.co.uk/wiki/CFS/ME_support_organisations

The notes that follow represent a summary of the rules for obtaining these benefits and of the benefits themselves. Please do seek help – see Useful documents and points of contact below and repeated in the Useful sources section (page 303).

Also, do be sure to be up to date with the new NICE Guideline on ME/CFS – NG206.[2] The ME Association has produced a useful summary.[3] This Guideline can help because it has recommendations in relation to needs assessments and social care.

The problem for CFS, ME and LC sufferers

The two main UK state welfare benefits for sufferers – Employment Support Allowance (ESA) and Personal Independent Payment (PIP), which has superseded Disability Living Allowance (DLA) – are 'scored' as to whether one qualifies or not, depending on answers to such questions as 'How far can you move safely and repeatedly on level ground without needing to stop?' (ESA50 form (the form for Work Capability Assessment) question 1 of Part 1 Physical Capability).

https://assets.publishing.service.gov.uk/government/uploads/system/uploads/attachment_data/file/975770/esa50-capability-for-work-questionnaire.pdf

To claim PIP, there is a different form asking about how your disability affects your ability to carry out everyday tasks – the latest copy of that form is PIP2.

https://assets.publishing.service.gov.uk/government/uploads/system/uploads/attachment_data/file/713118/pip2-how-your-disability-affects-you-form.pdf

However, whichever form you are filling in, the same problems as noted below will affect you.

The questions, and others that follow on Mental Capability for ESA, are more directed to conditions that are 'easier' to explain. Such questions are very difficult to answer adequately for conditions like CFS, ME and LC, which are so variable. A sufferer may be able to walk 50 metres in the morning but then that would require an hour's rest and then in the afternoon, that same sufferer might be bedridden. The next day they may be unable to walk even 10 metres, or even at all. (Please do see below regarding the DWP definition of 'moving' which is broader than just 'walking'.)

This problem is compounded by a feature of CFS, ME and LC sufferers that is almost universal in my experience – they are wildly optimistic about their own capabilities.

A worse (but more lovely) adjusted bunch of people you could hardly wish to meet! They want to get back to working life because they all miss it so much. So, they tend to overestimate what they can do. This is, in some ways, a good mindset, although it can lead to 'over-doing' things, which is problematic, but at least it means that there are very rarely motivational problems for engaging with me about what to do to get better. However, in terms of filling in the state welfare forms, this mindset is detrimental to giving a fair picture of the sufferer's actual level of disability.

So, in general terms, when filling in these forms, please do consider the guidelines in the section below.

General guidelines for filling in forms for ESA/PIP (and its legacy benefit, DLA) – 15 'rules'

'Rule' #1: Do take your time to explain your answers in detail

This means, for example, with regards to the above question on 'moving', do say that on some days you can walk this far, whereas, on other days you can only walk this far, and that on some days, you can't do any walking at all. Also mention the effects on your symptoms that such 'walking' would have and how long the recovery periods would be. Importantly, the DWP defines 'moving' to include any form of 'mobilisation' and so moving by wheelchair is included – please see point 14 below regarding the definition of 'mobilising'. So, your answers to this question may be to do with how far you can 'self-wheel' a wheelchair and the effect that such self-wheeling would have on symptoms. And also, do remember that this question, for example, asks about level ground – do read the questions *very* carefully.

It is ironic, in the extreme, that the people who deserve these benefits the most are probably the least able to complete the forms because they are so ill and so don't have the energy to give full answers. If you need help in completing the forms, do ask. The DWP can provide help as can the wonderful UK ME & Chronic Illness Benefits Advice Group's Facebook page

www.facebook.com/groups/278260135547189/

and also see below in 'Useful documents and points of contact'.

The Citizens' Advice Bureau may also be able to help or perhaps signpost you to where help can be found.

'Rule' #2: Always make sure that you include details of your 'worst days'

See below for comments on being able to 'consistently' perform tasks. You must let the DWP know just how bad you can be. Do use extra sheets to make sure that a full explanation is given.

'Rule' #3: Be clear and thorough about pain

If you cannot perform any of the tasks listed on the forms because of pain, make sure you state this in your answers.

'Rule' #4: Be clear about the need to rest

If you find a task so tiring that you cannot repeat it, or can only do it very slowly, explain this. Say how often you need to rest, how many times you could do the task, the symptoms you would experience during the task and afterwards and for how long afterwards.

'Rule' #5: Explain fully the variability of your condition

This may mean writing a new separate section, not specifically asked for in the forms. Talk about relapses and what causes them and how long they last for. Talk about how your condition varies from day to day, and from hour to hour. Remember all these things effectively mean that you cannot be 'relied upon' to work consistently.

'Rule' #6: Read the report on Fluctuating Conditions from the ME Association[4]

This report was produced by charities representing patients suffering with conditions such as MS, Parkinson's and ME. Take especial note of these important definitions of key terms. These are 'reliably', 'repeatedly' and 'safely', which should be applied to whether someone is judged capable of a particular task. If a claimant can't do a task reliably, repeatedly and safely, then they *cannot* do the task. Definitions taken from this report for performing a task are:

> '**Reliably** should mean completing a task to a satisfactory standard each time it is undertaken, within a reasonable amount of time – examples could be given to support this judgement.'
>
> '**Repeatedly** should mean being able to complete the task at a rate/frequency that is relevant to a workplace situation, without experiencing fatigue and/or pain, in line with what would be necessary for work. Guidance on how to define this should be given for each descriptor. For example, 'repeatedly' in terms of manual dexterity tasks, such as picking up a pound coin, may mean every few minutes or picking up several coins in a row, whereas 'repeatedly' mobilising 200m would mean the ability to do this several times in a day.'
>
> '**Safely** means that the task can be completed without risk to either the claimant, another employee, or someone else that the claimant comes in contact with.'

Stress all these factors when answering questions and always look to the variability and severity of your illness.

'Rule' #7: Consider for long you can 'consistently' and 'effectivley' perform any task

Can you consistently perform these tasks and do so 'effectively' over, say, a 16-hour week? Can you do this for weeks and months on end and be a 'reliable' employee? You have to be hard on yourself and brutally honest about these things. Also, remember that it is isn't 'just' 16 hours of work a week – there are the hours to get to and from work and the need to cook yourself breakfast, get dressed for work and so on. You must factor all these other requirements into the calculation as to whether you can actually *sustain* a working life.

'Rule' #8: Make sure that you explain how CFS, ME or LC affects your wider life

This means, not just the narrow questions that are asked on the forms. Use extra sheets if necessary to get your points across. Maybe describe an 'average day'. This is very difficult for such a variable condition, but it may help to give an overview of your condition.

'Rule' #9: Think about your ability to perform these tasks in a 'work-setting'

By a 'work setting', we mean with bright lights, lots of noise, perhaps quite a frenetic atmosphere with sudden and extra demands being possibly made on you at any time. Mention all your symptoms, using extra sheets if necessary.

'Rule' #10: Do always include 'payback' for any effort

Do stress, always, the symptoms that you can expect to experience as a consequence of performing a certain task. 'Payback' needs to be explained in detail as this is so specific to CFS, ME and LC. It is often misunderstood and so needs to be put across as well as you can.

'Rule' #11: Include any cognitive impairments

If you have cognitive impairments, then do mention these too. It is probably 'easiest' to put these points in the Mental Capability part of the forms. Do stress that these impairments do not arise from a mental illness but are as a result of your CFS, ME or LC.

'Rule' #12:-Include any separate medical conditions

However, if you do have other medical conditions, make sure that you include full details of these too.

'Rule' #13: Try to have letters of support from healthcare professionals who know you.

I can provide such letters and my patients have found them to be very helpful in securing the correct benefits and also the correct level of benefits. These support letters could be from anyone who knows your medical condition – GP, hospital consultant, nurse, physiotherapist etc. I have found that including test results to back up the symptomatology has been very useful – I include the Bell CFS Ability Scale with my letters of support and give an estimate of where the claimant is on that scale – see Appendix 5.

'Rule' #14: Be clear regarding the definition of 'mobility'

Remember that 'mobility' for the DWP is about whether you can 'get around', not *how* you get around, and so using a wheelchair to move 50 metres means that you are capable of 'mobilising' 50 metres. So, if you use a wheelchair, talk about the limitations of that too – how tired do you get, whether you need to be pushed, what your symptoms are like after 'self-wheeling' yourself etc.? Do you suffer from POTS if upright?

'Rule' #15: Keep copies of everything!

Make sure you photocopy everything you send to the DWP and also that you send it with a proof of posting and by a means that requires a signature at the other end so that you can track it.

Face-to-face assessments

You may be asked for a 'medical' or face-to-face assessment so that the DWP can assess your capabilities more 'directly'. Sometimes now they make use of phone and video calls for all types of assessment. The same 'rules' as above apply.

Make sure that you complete the section on the form concerning face-to-face assessments fully – state what help you would need to attend such an assessment, or even state that this would be impossible for you and that you therefore request a home visit, should a face-to-face assessment be required.

If you are called for a face-to-face assessment, always go with a friend for support. You may be able to ask for the assessment to be recorded – you could cite your poor memory or cognitive ability quite justifiably as a reason for wanting it recorded.

Some of the points that have arisen from personal experience from these face-to-face assessments are:

- You may be asked how you got there. This is not a 'nicety'; it is part of the assessment. If you say that you drove there then you may well be judged capable of driving even though, 'normally', you can't drive, or even that you may take a couple of days to recover from this.
- Ladies are sometimes complemented on their hair, or make-up, or fashion; this is again part of the assessment. 'You can't be that ill if you can look this good!' I would advise that you make no 'special effort' to look good for the face-to-face assessment – go as you normally are.
- Strength of handshake on meeting has even been used as a way of assessing someone.
- Treat every single part of the assessment as though you are being assessed because you are!

Appeals

Should you be denied benefits, then do follow the guidance that the DWP will send to you as to how to appeal. Again, obtain more supporting evidence and argue your case as above. I write letters of support for appeals and do have good success rates. As of June 2023, the www.benefitsandwork.co.uk website reported the following success rates for appeals and so it is well worth doing:

PIP: 68%

DLA: 59%

ESA: 50%

Isn't it astonishing that so many 'initial' decisions are incorrect? The stress and financial hardship that this puts sick and disabled people, and their families, through is a disgrace.

How the process may affect you

It is a really quite depressing process having to explain in black and white just how ill you are, but it is a necessary one. Be prepared for these feelings. It is also a physically demanding process for some sufferers to complete the forms within the deadlines. Again, do ask for help with this if you feel you need it. As I have said, the Citizens' Advice Bureau may be able to help or signpost you to where help is available. Remember that you deserve these benefits and so do carry on the fight, if necessary. See also below and the Useful Resources section.

Details of ESA and PIP and Attendance and Carers' Allowance

1. Employment Support Allowance (ESA)

This is a benefit paid to people who are not able to work. Please see:

www.gov.uk/employment-support-allowance/overview

Also see:

www.citizensadvice.org.uk/benefits/sick-or-disabled-people-and-carers/employment-and-support-allowance/while-youre-getting-esa/about-the-esa-groups/

This gives the differences between the two main types of ESA, which are as follows – if you're eligible for ESA, you'll be put into either:

a. the Support Group.
b. the Work-Related Activity Group.

The Support Group

If you've been put in the Support Group, it means the DWP has decided that you can't work and that it doesn't expect you to do anything to improve your chances of finding work. However, if you're in this group and decide that you want to take part in work-related activity anyway, you can do so. Use the contact details on your decision letter to let the DWP know you want to do this. They'll let you know if there's any suitable work-related activity going on in your area that you can join.

The Work-Related Activity Group

If you've been put into the Work-Related Activity Group, it means the DWP has decided that your disability or health condition does limit your ability to work right now, but that there are things you can do to improve this. You're not expected to look for work, but you can be asked to go to a work-focused interview and then do work-related activities. These activities are things that the DWP thinks will improve your chances of working in the future.

You won't need to go to a work-focused interview or do any work-related activities if:

a. you're a single parent with a child under one year old.
b. you've reached Pension Credit age.

The rates (April 2023) are as follows: [https://www.gov.uk/employment-support-allowance/what-youll-get]

You'll normally get the assessment rate for 13 weeks after your claim. This will be:

- up to £67.20 a week if you're aged under 25
- up to £84.80 a week if you're aged 25 or over

After that, if you're entitled to ESA, you'll be placed in one of two groups and will receive:

- up to £84.80 a week if you're in the work-related activity group
- up to £129.50 a week if you're in the support group.

There is also a further sub-division of ESA into Contribution-based and Income-related:

- **Contribution-based** (or 'Contributory') ESA is paid if you have paid enough National Insurance contributions. You can get it even if your partner works or if you have savings:
    - Contribution-based ESA entitlement is limited to one year from the time entitlement began for those in the Work-Related Activity Group.
    - For those in the Support Group, there is no time limit for Contribution-based ESA.
- **Income-related** ESA is payable if you have not paid enough National Insurance contributions. Income-related ESA has no time limit and can be claimed for as long as you meet the qualifying criteria. The qualifying criteria for Income-related ESA can be quite complex but essentially, if your savings are less than £16,000 (at the time of going to press) and if you have a partner or civil partner who works for less than 24 hours a week on average, then you should qualify:

www.entitledto.co.uk/help/eligibility-employment-and-support-allowance

There have been further complications with the introduction of Universal Credit (UC) – in particular, 'new style' ESA. In plain terms, 'old-style' ESA is 'ESA awarded' (i.e. using the ESA50 WCA form as above) and paid outside the UC system, as described above. It can comprise both Contribution-based ESA and Income-related ESA. By contrast, 'new style' ESA is 'ESA awarded' and paid under the UC system.

Contact for ESA

Telephone: 0800 055 6688
Textphone: 0800 328 1344
Relay UK (if you cannot hear or speak on the phone): 18001 then 0800 055 6688
Website: www.gov.uk/employment-support-allowance/how-to-claim

2. Personal Independence Payment (PIP)

This is a benefit paid to people to help with the costs of being long-term ill or disabled. How much you will receive will depend on how your illness affects you, not on the illness itself – please see:- www.gov.uk/pip/overview

PIP is usually paid every four weeks. It's tax free and you can get it whether you're in or out of work.

It's made up of two components (parts). One part is the Daily Living Component and assesses your needs for help with everyday tasks; the other is the Mobility Component and this looks at your needs associated with poor mobility. Whether you get one or both of these depends on how your condition affects you. Rates at the time of going to press are:

Daily Living component	**Weekly rate**
Standard	£68.10
Enhanced	£101.75
Mobility component	**Weekly rate**
Standard	£26.90
Enhanced	£71.00

PIP is available for those aged over 16.

You must also be under State Pension Age if you've not received PIP before.

Contact for PIP

Telephone: 0800 121 4433
Textphone: 0800 121 4493
Relay UK (if you cannot hear or speak on the phone): 18001 then 0800 121 4433
Website: www.gov.uk/disability-benefits-helpline

3. Attendance Allowance (AA)

You could get AA (www.gov.uk/attendance-allowance/overview) at £68.10 or £101.75 a week (at the time of going to press) to help with personal care because you're physically or mentally disabled and you've reached State Pension Age. It's paid at two different rates and how much you get depends on the level of care that you need because of your disability.

The other benefits you get can increase if you get Attendance Allowance.

Contact for AA

Telephone: 0800 731 0122
Textphone: 0800 731 0317
Relay UK (if you cannot hear or speak on the phone): 18001 then 0800 731 0122
Website: www.gov.uk/attendance-allowance/how-to-claim

4. Carers' Allowance (CA)

CA is a benefit paid to someone who cares for someone else who is ill or disabled. In general terms:

- You could get £76.75 a week (at the time of going to press) if you care for someone for at least 35 hours a week and they get 'certain benefits'.
- You don't have to be related to, or live with, the person you care for.
- You won't be paid extra if you care for more than one person.

The 'certain benefits' mentioned above are:

- Personal Independence Payment (PIP – Daily Living component)
- Disability Living Allowance (legacy) (the middle or highest care rate)

- Attendance Allowance (AA)
- Constant Attendance Allowance at or above the normal maximum rate with an Industrial Injuries Disablement Benefit
- Constant Attendance Allowance at the basic (full day) rate with a War Disablement Pension
- Armed Forces Independence Payment
- Child Disability Payment: the middle or highest care rate
- Adult Disability Payment: the daily living component at the standard or enhanced rate

Contact for CA

Telephone: 0800 731 0297
Textphone: 0800 731 0317
Relay UK (if you cannot hear or speak on the phone): 18001 then 0800 731 0297
Website: www.gov.uk/carers-allowance/how-to-claim

Useful documents and points of contact

- Fluctuating Conditions Report: www.meassociation.org.uk/wp-content/uploads/Fluctuating_conditions_report_FINAL.pdf
- DWP webpages on ESA: www.gov.uk/employment-support-allowance/overview
- CAB webpages on ESA: www.citizensadvice.org.uk/benefits/sick-or-disabled-people-and-carers/employment-and-support-allowance/while-youre-getting-esa/about-the-esa-groups/
- DWP webpages on PIP: www.gov.uk/pip/overview
- DWP webpages on AA: www.gov.uk/attendance-allowance/overview
- DWP webpages on CA: www.gov.uk/carers-allowance/overview
- UK ME & Chronic Illness Benefits Advice Facebook group (highly recommended!) www.facebook.com/groups/278260135547189/
- Benefits and Welfare website: www.benefitsandwork.co.uk/

The mission statement of this website on its Home Page is as follows:

'Get the benefits you're entitled to.

Don't lose out just because the system isn't fair.

For 20 years, our guides, training, forum and newsletters have helped thousands of claimants, carers and their support workers to make the best possible claims and appeals.

Join the Benefits and Work community to get the correct award of PIP, ESA, UC or DLA.'

It provides up-to-date information about the best way to apply for and appeal all UK welfare benefits. Details of how to subscribe are included on its 'Join us' page. It costs £19.95 (at the time of going to press) for an annual subscription.

- The ME Association produces *excellent* guides to help you through the process of filling in the ESA, PIP and DLA forms and also how to appeal: Please see: https://meassociation.org.uk/product-category/benefits/ for the full list of guides.

Other benefits

Do check your eligibility for other benefits such as:

- Universal Credit: www.gov.uk/universal-credit
- Housing Benefit: www.gov.uk/housing-benefit
- Working and Child Tax Credits (replaced by Universal Credit but see here for legacy benefits): www.gov.uk/claim-tax-credits
- Pension Credit: www.gov.uk/pension-credit
- Council Tax Reduction: www.gov.uk/apply-council-tax-reduction
- Applying for a Needs Assessment by Social Services: www.gov.uk/apply-needs-assessment-social-services
- …and others, including reduced rates for internet access etc available from private companies such as BT.

Postscript – UK government consultation

As of September 2023, the UK Government launched another consultation on welfare benefits, running until 30 October 2023. This is entirely separate from, and additional to, the Spring 2023 White Paper as discussed at the start of this chapter. This new consultation takes as its starting point the idea that working practices have changed since the Covid pandemic and that many more people now work from home. Therefore, the consultation looks at key areas that used to confer entitlement to certain benefits and asks the question whether these areas should still be seen as a 'block' to seeking employment. These areas are:

- Mobilising – the argument here is that if one is working at home, then there is no need to be able to 'mobilise' (walk or self-propel a wheelchair).
- Controlling your bowels and bladder – the argument here is that if one is at home then one can always deal with one's toilet needs in privacy.
- Coping with social engagement – the argument here is that if one is working from home, then social anxiety is not a factor.
- Getting about – the argument here is that one does not need to be able to get about if one is working from home – 'getting about' issues include physical problems and mental health problems such as agoraphobia.

According to the consultation document, any changes will be legislated on in 2024 and come into force in 2025 – after the next General Election.

The changes, if enacted, would affect new claimants from 2025 and existing claimants when their award is reviewed from 2025 onwards.

With future reprints of this book we will endeavour to keep the details listed up-to-date.

Appendix 5

The Bell CFS Ability Scale – a measure of where you are

Introduction

The fatigue in CFS, ME and LC is both mental and physical. For some sufferers, the physical is the greatest burden and for others, the mental fatigue is most troublesome. The Bell CFS Ability Scale was developed by Dr David Bell[1] as a clinically useful way to assess response to treatment – it combines physical and mental activity with levels of wellness. This is not entirely satisfactory because different people suffer in different ways, but it does give an idea of the overall level of disability.

There are many other scales/questionnaires used to assess the level of ability among CFS/ME sufferers. It is an area of much debate and a detailed discussion is beyond the scope of this book, but interested readers can start here, if they are motivated to do so: https://me-pedia.org/wiki/Questionnaires_and_tools_to_assess_ME/CFS_symptoms_or_severity

Briefly, some scales are better suited when one is doing research, and some are more suited for clinical situations. Some patients groups do not like the fact that some (clinically-based) scales focus on pain, fatigue and *overall* disability and would prefer scales that look at the constellation of symptoms found in CFS and ME, and cite, for example, the International Consensus Criteria, which can be found on my website.[2]

Above all, I am a clinician and whilst I do accept that the International Consensus Criteria represent a more complete picture of the symptom load of CFS and ME sufferers, I see my job as reducing the overall level of disability of my patients and increasing their functionality and in so doing improving their quality of life. In a nutshell, my job, as a clinician, is to help them get better! The Bell Scale is a good clinical scale and does help me monitor and understand my patients' overall 'health', and therefore it has been the one that I have used, and continue to use, in my practice.

The scale

100: No symptoms with exercise. Normal overall activity. Able to work or do house/homework full time with no difficulty.

90: No symptoms at rest. Mild symptoms with physical activity. Normal overall activity level. Able to work full time without difficulty.

80: Mild symptoms at rest. Symptoms worsened by exertion. Minimal activity restriction needed for activities requiring exertion only. Able to work full time but with difficulty in jobs requiring exertion.

70: Mild symptoms at rest. Some daily activity limitation clearly noted. Overall functioning close to 90% of expected except for activities requiring exertion. Able to work/do housework full time with difficulty. Need to rest during the day.

60: Mild to moderate symptoms at rest. Daily activity limitation clearly noted. Overall functioning 70% to 90%. Unable to work full time in jobs requiring physical labour (including just standing), but able to work full time in light activity (sitting) if hours are flexible.

50: Moderate symptoms at rest. Moderate to severe symptoms with exercise or activity; overall activity level reduced to 70% of expected. Unable to perform strenuous duties, but able to perform light duties or deskwork for 4-5 hours a day, but requires rest periods. Has to rest/sleep 1-2 hours daily.

40: Moderate symptoms at rest. Moderate to severe symptoms with exercise or activity. Overall activity level reduced to 50-70% of expected. Able to go out once or twice a week. Unable to perform strenuous duties. Able to work sitting down at home 3-4 hours a day but requires rest periods.

30: Moderate to severe symptoms at rest. Severe symptoms with any exercise. Overall activity level reduced to 50% of expected. Usually confined to house.

Unable to perform any strenuous tasks. Able to perform deskwork 2-3 hours a day but requires rest periods.

20: Moderate to severe symptoms at rest. Unable to perform strenuous activity. Overall activity 30-50% of expected. Unable to leave house except rarely. Confined to bed most of day. Unable to concentrate for more than 1 hour a day.

10: Severe symptoms at rest. Bedridden the majority of the time. No travel outside of the house. Marked cognitive symptoms preventing concentration.

0: Severe symptoms on a continuous basis. Bedridden constantly, unable to care for self.

Please, note that 'desk work' includes everyday tasks such as sitting at a table to eat or read.

References

Chapter 1: The road map for recovery

1. NICE Guideline [NG206] on ME/CFS. National Institute for Health and Care Excellence, UK. www.nice.org.uk/guidance/ng206/chapter/Recommendations#managing-mecfs (accessed 1 October 2023)
2. Kindlon T. Reporting of Harms Associated with Graded Exercise Therapy and Cognitive Behavioural Therapy in Myalgic Encephalomyelitis/Chronic Fatigue Syndrome. *Bulletin of the IACFS/ME* 2011; 19(2): 59-11. www.researchgate.net/publication/216572185_Reporting_of_Harms_Associated_with_Graded_Exercise_Therapy_and_Cognitive_Behavioural_Therapy_in_Myalgic_EncephalomyelitisChronic_Fatigue_Syndrome
3. Geraghty K, Hann M, Kurtev S. Myalgic encephalomyelitis/chronic fatigue syndrome patients' reports of symptom changes following cognitive behavioural therapy, graded exercise therapy and pacing treatments: Analysis of a primary survey compared with secondary surveys. *Journal of Health Psychology* 2017; 24(10). doi: 10.1177/1359105317726152 http://journals.sagepub.com/eprint/hWSxVIBTzDtqisvafkhE/full

Chapter 2: CFS – the symptoms of poor energy delivery

1. Peckerman A, LaManca JL, Dahl KA, et al. Abnormal impedance cardiography predicts symptom severity in chronic fatigue syndrome. *Am J Med Sci* 2003; 326(2): 55-60. doi: 10.1097/00000441-200308000-00001. https://pubmed.ncbi.nlm.nih.gov/12920435/
2. VanElzakker MB. Chronic fatigue syndrome from vagus nerve infection: a psychoneuroimmunological hypothesis. *Med Hypotheses* 2013; 81(3): 414-423. https://pubmed.ncbi.nlm.nih.gov/23790471/

Chapter 3: The mechanisms of poor energy delilvery and how to treat them

1. Myhill S. 5G – the What, the Why and the How. Updated February 2023 with a comment by Michael Mansfield KC. www.drmyhill.co.uk/wiki/5G_%E2%80%93_the_WHAT_the_WHY_and_the_HOW (accessed 20 October 2023)

Chapter 4: First steps

1. Bristol Stool Chart. https://en.wikipedia.org/wiki/Bristol_stool_scale (accessed 14 October 2023)
2. Burkitt D. *Don't Forget Fibre in your Diet* Harper Collins; 1979. www.amazon.co.uk/Dont-Forget-Fibre-Your-Diet/dp/0906348072/
3. Bredesen D. Reversal of cognitive decline: A novel therapeutic program. 2014 www.drmyhill.co.uk/drmyhill/images/0/07/Reversal-of-Cognitive-decline-Bredesen.pdf
4. Glenn Gibson Profile. Dept of Food and Nutrition Sciences, University of Reading. www.reading.ac.uk/food/about/staff/g-r-gibson.aspx (accessed 14 October 2023)
5. Biser JA. Really wild remedies – Medicinal Plant Use by Animals. *Zoogoer* Jan-Feb 1998 https://web.archive.org/web/20040630010109/http://nationalzoo.si.edu/Publications/Zoogoer/1998/1/reallywildremedies.cfm

Chapter 5: It's mitochondria not hypochondria

1. Myhill S, Booth N, McLaren-Howard J. Chronic fatigue syndrome and mitochondrial dysfunction. *International Journal of Clinical and Experimental Medicine* 2009; 2: 1-16 www.ncbi.nlm.nih.gov/pmc/articles/PMC2680051/.
2. Booth N, Myhill S, McLaren-Howard J. Mitochondrial dysfunction and pathophysiology of myalgic encephalomyelitis/chronic fatigue syndrome (ME/CFS). *International Journal of Clinical and Experimental Medicine* 2012; 5(3): 208-220 www.ncbi.nlm.nih.gov/pmc/articles/PMC3403556
3. Myhill S, Booth NE, McLaren-Howard J. Targeting mitochondrial dysfunction in the treatment of myalgic encephalomyelitis/chronic fatigue syndrome (ME/CFS) – a clinical audit. *International Journal of Clinical and Experimental Medicine* 2013; 6(1): 1-15. www.ncbi.nlm.nih.gov/pmc/articles/PMC3515971
4. Peckerman A, Dahl KA, Chemitiganti R, et al. Abnormal Impedance Cardiography Predicts

Symptom Severity in Chronic Fatigue Syndrome. *American Journal of the Medical Sciences* 2003; 326(2):55-60. www.amjmedsci.com/article/S0002-9629(15)34232-4/fulltext
5. Norman Booth's publications: www.researchgate.net/profile/Norman-Booth-2 plus Norman gave great support to OMEGA – The Oxford ME Group for Action – which is still very active: https://omegaoxon.org
6. 5G – the What, the Why and the How. Updated February 2023 with a comment by Michael Mansfield KC. www.drmyhill.co.uk/wiki/5G_%E2%80%93_the_WHAT_the_WHY_and_the_HOW (accessed 20 October 2023)
7. Pollack G. *Fourth Phase of Water: Beyond Solid, Liquid & Vapor: Beyond Solid, Liquid, and Vapor.* Ebner & Sons; 2013. www.amazon.co.uk/Fourth-Phase-Water-Beyond-Liquid/dp/0962689548

Chapter 6: Oxygen

1. Geena Davis Institute on Gender in Media. The Scully Effect: I want to believe in STEM. https://seejane.org/research-informs-empowers/the-scully-effect-i-want-to-believe-in-stem (accessed 23 October 2023)
2. Iowa Head and Neck Protocols. Pulse oximetry basic principles and interpretation. 10 March 2017. https://medicine.uiowa.edu/iowaprotocols/pulse-oximetry-basic-principles-and-interpretation (accessed 23 October 2023)

Chapter 7: The thyroid accelerator pedal and the adrenal gearbox

1. ME Research UK. CFS/ME in women and men. 19 August 2015. www.meresearch.org.uk/sex-differences-in-mecfs (accessed 23 October 2023)
2. Arafah BM. Increased Need for Thyroxine in Women with Hypothyroidism during Estrogen Therapy. *N Engl J Med* 2001; 344: 1743-1749. https://pubmed.ncbi.nlm.nih.gov/11396440/
3. Panicker V. Genetics of Thyroid Function and Disease. *Clin Biochem Rev* 2011; 32(4): 165–175. www.ncbi.nlm.nih.gov/ pmc/articles/PMC3219766/
4. Surks M. Lithium and the Thyroid. www.uptodate.com/ contents/lithium-and-the-thyroid
5. Loh K-C. Amiodarone-induced thyroid disorders: a clinical review. *BMJ* 76(893) https://pmj.bmj.com/ content/76/893/133
6. Bax ND, Lennard MA, Tucker GT. Effect of beta blockers on thyroid hormone. *BMJ* 1980;

281(6250): 1283. doi: 10.1136/bmj.281.6250.1283

7. Vera-Lastra O, Navarro AO, Domiguez MPC, et al. Two Cases of Graves' Disease Following SARS-CoV-2 Vaccination: An Autoimmune/Inflammatory Syndrome Induced by Adjuvants. *Thyroid* 2021; 31(9): 1436-1439. doi: 10.1089/thy.2021.0142 https://pubmed.ncbi.nlm.nih.gov/33858208/
8. Nishihara E, Ohye H, Amino N, et al. Clinical Characteristics of 852 Patients with Subacute Thyroiditis before Treatment. *Internal Medicine* 2008; 47(8): 725-729. doi: 10.2169/internalmedicine.47.0740 www.jstage.jst.go.jp/article/internalmedicine/47/8/47_8_725/_article

Chapter 8: Sleep – when healing and repair take place

1. Halberg F, Cornelissen G, Katinas G, et al. Transdisciplinary unifying implications of circadian findings in the 1950s. *Journal of Circadian Rhythms* 2003; 1: Art 2. doi: 10.1186/1740-3391-1-2 www.jcircadianrhythms.com/articles/10.1186/1740-3391-1-2/
2. Boke of St Albans. Internet Archive. https://archive.org/stream/bokeofsaintalban00bern/bokeofsaintalban00bern_djvu.txt
3. Burwell CS, Robin ED, Whaley RD, Bickelmann AG. Extreme obesity associated with alveolar hypoventilation-a Pickwickian syndrome. *Am J Med* 1956; 21: 811- 818. www.sciencedirect.com/science/article/pii/0002934356900948
4. Nishihara K. Disclosure of the major causes of mental illness—mitochondrial deterioration in brain neurons via opportunistic infection. *Journal of Biological Physics and Chemistry* 2012; 12: 11-18. www.drmyhill.co.uk/drmyhill/images/d/dc/NISHIHARA.pdf

Chapter 9: Pacing and the right sort of exercise

1. Baker R. Lecture notes. https://courses.maths.ox.ac.uk/pluginfile.php/12132/mod_resource/content/2/FurtherMathematicalBiologyNotes2021.pdf
2. McGuff D, Little J. Body by Science: a research-based programme for strength training, body building and complete fitness in 12 minutes a week. McGraw-Hill Education; 2009. www.amazon.co.uk/Body-Science-Research-Strength-Training/dp/0071597174/

Chapter 10: Myalgic encephalitis and long covid – the symptoms of inflammation

1. Wong T, Weitzer D. Long COVID and Myalgic Encephalomyelitis/Chronic Fatigue

Syndrome (ME/CFS) – A Systemic Review and Comparison of Clinical Presentation and Symptomatology. *Medicina (Kaunas)* 2021; 57(5): 418. https://pubmed.ncbi.nlm.nih.gov/33925784/

Chapter 13: The general approach to reducing inflammation

1. National Fire Chiefs Council (NFCC). www.ukfrs.com/modal/general-cm/13785/313689/document/nojs [this link doesn't work?]
2. Berg RD. Bacterial translocation from the gastrointestinal tract. *Adv Exp Med* 1999; 473: 11-30. https://pubmed.ncbi.nlm.nih.gov/10659341/
3. Myhill S. Probiotics – we should all be taking these all the time. February 2022. www.drmyhill.co.uk/wiki/Probiotics_-_we_should_all_be_taking_these_all_the_time_and_double_the_dose_following_antibiotics_and_gastroenteritis
4. Myhill S. Faecal bacteriotherapy. October 2022. www.drmyhill.co.uk/wiki/Faecal_bacteriotherapy

4A. Borody TJ, Nowak A, Finlayson S. The GI microbiome and its role in chronic fatigue syndrome: A summary of bacteriotherapy. *J Australas Coll Nutr Environ Med* 2012; 31(3): 3-8. https://search.informit.org/doi/10.3316/INFORMIT.119626231492520

5. Myhill S. B12 – the rationale for using B12 in CFS. March 2022. www.drmyhill.co.uk/wiki/B12_-_rationale_for_using_vitamin_B12_in_CFS
6. Ingraham C. *Help Your Dog Heal Itself.* Ingraham Trading Ltd; 2018. www.amazon.co.uk/Help-Your-Dog-Heal-Itself/dp/0952482746/
7. Pizzorno L. Nothing boring about boron. *Integr Med (Encinitas)* 2015; 14(4): 35-48. www.ncbi.nlm.nih.gov/pmc/articles/PMC4712861/
8. https://ldnresearchtrust.org/

Chapter 14: Detoxing

1. Peckham S, Awosefo N. Water Fluoridation: A Critical Review of the Physiological Effects of Ingested Fluoride as a Public Health Intervention. *Scientific World Journal* 2014; 2014: 293019. doi: 10.1155/2014/293019
2. Gregory AE, Titball R, Williamson D. Vaccine delivery using nanoparticles. *Front Cell Infect Microbiol* 2013; 3: 13. doi: 10.3389/fcimb.2013.00013
3. Myhill S. Mercury. www.drmyhill.co.uk/wiki/Mercury_-_Toxicity_of_Dental_Amalgam_-_Why_you_should_have_your_dental_amalgams_removed (Accessed 15 August 2023)
4. Guo J-Y, Zeng EY, Wu F-C, et al. Organochlorine pesticides in seafood products from

southern China and health risk assessment. *Environ Toxicol Chem* 2007; 26(6): 1109-1115. doi: 10.1897/06-446r.1

5. Myhill S. 5G – the What, the Why and the How. Updated February 2023 with a comment by Michael Mansfield KC. www.drmyhill.co.uk/wiki/5G_–_the_WHAT_the_WHY_and_the_HOW (accessed 15 August 2023)
6. Formuzis A. EWG's "Dirty Dozen" list of hormone-disrupting chemicals. 28 October 2013. www.ewg.org/news-insights/news-release/ewgs-dirty-dozen-list-hormone-disrupting-chemicals (Accessed 15 August 2023)
7. Negi S, Bala L, Chopra D, et al. Tattoo inks are toxicological risks to human health: A systematic review of their ingredients, fate inside skin, toxicity due to polycyclic aromatic hydrocarbons, primary aromatic amines, metals, and overview of regulatory frameworks. *Toxicol Ind Health* 2022; 38(7): 417-434. doi: 10.1177/07482337221100870
8. Lehner K, Santarelli F, Vasold R, et al. Black tattoo inks are a source of problematic substances such as dibutyl phthalate. *Contact Dermatitis* 2011; 65(4): 231-238. doi: 10.1111/j.1600-0536.2011.01947.x
9. Mesnage R, Ano M, Costanzo M, et al. Transcriptome profile analysis reflects rat liver and kidney damage following chronic ultra-low dose Roundup exposure. *Environmental Health* 2015; 14: 70. doi: 10.1186/s12940-015-0056-1
10. Myhill S. Silicone breast implants. www.drmyhill.co.uk/wiki/Silicone_Breast_Implants_and_Injections (Accessed 15 August 2023)
11. Microplastics. www.nhm.ac.uk/discover/what-are-microplastics.html (Accessed 15 August 2023)
12. Rea WJ, Md YP, Faaem ARJD, et al. Reduction of chemical sensitivity by means of heat depuration, physical therapy and nutritional supplementation in a controlled environment. *Journal-of-Nutritional-and-Environmental-Medicine* 1996; 6(2): 141-148. doi: 10.3109/13590849609001042
13. Waring RH. Report on Absorption of magnesium sulfate (Epsom salts) across the skin. *The Magnesium Online Library* www.mgwater.com/transdermal.shtml (Accessed 15 August 2023)
14. Rackham H (trans). *Pliny's Natural History* Vol. 9. London: Heinemann, 1972: pp 285.

Chapter 15: The general approach to treating chronic infection

1. Itzhaki RF. Overwhelming Evidence for a Major Role for Herpes Simplex Virus Type 1 (HSV1) in Alzheimer's Disease (AD); Underwhelming Evidence against. *Vaccines* 2021; 9(6): 679. doi: 10.3390/vaccines9060679
2. Kaul M. HIV-1 associated dementia. *Current Opinion in Neurology* 2009; 22(3): 315-320. doi: 10.1097/WCO.0b013e328329cf3c

3. Kristofertitsch W, Aboulenein-Djamshidian F, Jecel J, et al. Secondary dementia due to Lyme neuroborreliosis, *Wien Klin Wochenschr* 2018; 130(15): 468-478. doi: 10.1007/s00508-018-1361-9
4. Sena G, Gallelli G. An increased severity of peripheral arterial disease in the COVID-19 era. *J Vasc Surgery* 2020; 72(2): 758. doi: 10.1016/j.jvs.2020.04.489
5. Karnoutsos K, Papastergiou P, Stefanidis S, Vakaloudi A. Periodontitis as a risk factor for cardiovascular disease: The role of anti-phosphorylcholine and anti-cardiolipin antibodies. *Hippokratia* 2008; 12(3): 144-149. www.ncbi.nlm.nih.gov/pmc/articles/PMC2504402/
6. de Souza CRT, Almeida MCA, Khayat AS, et al. Association between Helicobacter pylori, Epstein-Barr virus, human papillomavirus and gastric adenocarcinomas. *World J Gastroentrol* 2018; 24(43): 4928-4938. doi: 10.3748/wjg.v24.i43.4928
7. Benzie IFF, Wachtel-Galor S. *Herbal Medicine 2nd Edition: Biomolecular and Clinical Aspects, Oxidative Stress and Disease.* www.ncbi.nlm.nih.gov/books/NBK92771/
8. Lee C-Y, Nguyen AT, Doan LH, et al. Repurposing Astragalus Polysaccharide PG2 for Inhibiting ACE2 and SARS-CoV-2 Spike Syncytial Formation and Anti-Inflammatory Effects. *Viruses* 2023; 15(3): 641. doi: 10.3390/v15030641.
9. Verma AK. Cordycepin: a bioactive metabolite of C ordyceps militaris and polyadenylation inhibitor with therapeutic potential against COVID-19. *J Biomol Struct Dyn* 2022; 40(8): 3745-3752. doi: 10.1080/07391102.2020.1850352
10. Karosanidze I, Kiladze U, Kirtadze N, et al. Efficacy of Adaptogens in Patients with Long COVID-19: A Randomized, Quadruple-Blind, Placebo-Controlled Trial. *Pharmaceuticals* 2022; 15(3): 345. doi: 10.3390/ph15030345.
11. Xiong X, Wang P, Su K, Cho WC, Xing Y. Chinese herbal medicine for coronavirus disease 2019: A systematic review and meta-analysis. doi: 10.1016/j.phrs.2020.105056
12. The Last of Us Wiki. Cordyceps brain infection. https://thelastofus.fandom.com/wiki/Cordyceps_brain_infection (accessed 23 October 2023)
13. Yahaya MFZR, Alias Z, Karsani SA. Subtractive Protein Profiling of Salmonella typhimurium Biofilm Treated with DMSO. *Protein J* 2017; 36(4): 286-298. doi: 10.1007/s10930-017-9719-9.
14. Murav'ev IV, Loskutova TT, Anikina NV, et al. The effect of dimethyl sulfoxide on the thromboelastographic indices and the microcirculation in patients with rheumatic diseases. *Clinical Trials* 1989; 61(12): 106-109.
15. Get Fitt. Far Infrared Rays (FIR) Research. www.get-fitt.com/what_infrared_rays/research/ (Accessed 18 August 2023)
16. Wikipedia. Photodynamic therapy. https://en.wikipedia.org/wiki/Photodynamic_therapy (Accessed 18 August 2023)

Chapter 16: Dimethylsulphoxide (DMSO)

1. Charlson RJ, Lovelock JE, Andreae MO, Warren S. Oceanic phytoplankton, atmospheric sulphur, cloud albedo and climate. *Nature* 1987; 326(6114): 655-661.
2. Pollack G. *The Fourth Phase of Water: Beyond solid, liquid and vapor.* Ebner & Sons; 2013. www.amazon.co.uk/Fourth-Phase-Water-Beyond-Liquid/dp/0962689548
3. Huang S-H, Wu C-H, Chen S-J, et al. Immunomodulatory effects and potential clinical applications of dimethyl sulfoxide. *Immunobiology* 2020; 225(3): 151906. doi: 10.1016/j.imbio.2020.151906
4. Ashwood-Smith MJ. *The Radioprotective Action of Dimethyl Sulphoxide and Various Other Sulphoxides. International J Radiation Biology and Related Studies in Physics, Chemistry and Medicine* 1961; 3(1): 41-48. doi: 10.1080/09553006114550051
5. Walker M. *DMSO: Nature's Healer*. Avery Publishing Group; 1993
6. RxList. DMSO (Dimethylsulfoxide). www.rxlist.com/dmso_dimethylsulfoxide/supplements.htm (Accessed 18 August 2023)
7. Misidou C, Papagoras C. Complex regional pain syndrome: An update. *Mediterr J Rheumatol* 2019; 30(1): 16-25. doi: 10.31138/mjr.30.1.16
8. Sadananda G, Velmurugan JD, Subramaniam JR. DMSO Delays Alzheimer Disease Causing Aβ-induced Paralysis in C. elegans through Modulation of Glutamate/Acetylcholine Neurotransmission. *Ann Neurosci* 2021; 28(1-2): 55-64. doi: 10.1177/09727531211046369
9. Igimi H, Asakawa S, Tamura R, et al. DMSO preparation as a direct solubilizer of calcium bilirubinate stones. *Hepatogastroenterology* 1994; 41(1): 65-69. PMID: 8175120
10. Parcell S. Sulfur in human nutrition and applications in medicine. *Altern Med Rev* 2002; 7(1): 22-44. PMID: 11896744
11. Segura G. DMSO – The real miracle solution. *Precious Organics* 12 May 2011. www.preciousorganics.com.au/pages/dmso-the-real-miracle-solution (Accessed 19 August 2023)
12. Vollmer A. *Healing with DMSO: The complete guide to safe and natural treatments for managing pain, inflammation, and other chronic ailments with dimethyl sulfoxide.* Ulysses Press; 2020.

Chapter 17: Methylene blue for all chronic infections

1. BnF Catalogue general. https://catalogue.bnf.fr/rechercher.
2. Tucker D, Lu Y, Zhang Q. From mitochondrial function to neuroprotection – an emerging role for methylene blue. *Mol Neurobiol* 2018; 55(6): 5137-5153. doi: 10.1007/s12035-017-0712-2

3. Ginimuge PR, Jyothi SD. Methylene blue: Revisited. *J Anaesthesiol Clin Pharmacol* 2010; 26(4): 517-520. PMID: 21547182
4. Scigliano G, Scigliano GA. Methylene blue in covid-19. *Medical Hypotheses* 2021; 146: 110455. doi: 10.1016/j.mehy.2020.110455
5. Lu G, Nagbanshi M, Goldau N, et al. Efficacy and safety of methylene blue in the treatment of malaria: a systematic review. *BMC Med* 2018; 16(1): 59. doi: 10.1186/s12916-018-1045-3
6. Cagno V, Medaglia C, Cerny A, et al. Methylene Blue has a potent antiviral activity against SARS-CoV-2 and H1N1 influenza virus in the absence of UV-activation in vitro. *Nature: Scientific Reports* 2021; 11: 14295. doi: 10.1038/s41598-021-92481-9
7. Wood C, Habib N. Methylene blue therapy of viral disease. *United States Patient Application Publication* 23 November 2006. US 2006/0264423 A1. https://patentimages.storage.googleapis.com/de/67/80/359dcdc11bdf03/US20060264423A1.pdf
8. Hamidi-Alamdari D, Hafizi-Lotfabadi S, Bagheri-Moghaddam A, et al. Methylene blue for treatment of hospitalized covid-19 patients: A randomized, controlled, open-label clinical trial, Phase 2. *Rev Invest Clin* 2021; 73(3): 190-198. doi: 10.24875/RIC.21000028
9. Dabholkar N, Gorantla S, Dubey SK, et al. Repurposing methylene blue in the management of COVID-19: Mechanistic aspects and clinical investigations. *Biomedicine & Pharmacotherapy* 2021; 142: 112023. doi: 10.1016/j.biopha.2021.112023
10. Ansari MA, Fatima Z, Hameed S. Antifungal action of methylene blue involves mitochondrial dysfunction and disruption of redox and membrane homeostasis in C. albicans. *Open Microbiol J* 2016; 10: 12-22. doi: 10.2174/1874285801610010012
11. Coen J. Top 6 benefits of methylene blue and dosage side effects. SelfDecode. https://drugs.selfdecode.com/blog/methylene-blue-the-cheapest-cognitive-enhancer/ (Accessed 19 August 2023)
12. Naylor GJ, Smith AH, Connelly P. A controlled trial of methylene blue in severe depressive illness. *Biol Psychiatry* 1987; 22(5): 657-659. doi: 10.1016/0006-3223(87)90194-6
13. Delport A, Harvey BH, Petzer A, Petzer JP. Methylene blue and its analogues as antidepressant compounds. *Metab Brain Dis* 2017; 32(5): 1357-1382. doi: 10.1007/s11011-017-0081-6
14. AAPP. Monoamine Oxidase Inhibitors (MAOI): Significant Drug-Drug/Drug-Food Interactions with MAOIs. https://aapp.org/guideline/maoi/interactions (Accessed 19 August 2023)
15. MAO Inhibitors Inc. Serious risks with MAO inhibitors. https://maoinhibitors.com/serious-risks/ (Accessed 19 August 2023)
16. Levy TE. Resolving colds to advance COVID with methylene blue. *Orthomolecular Medicine News Service* 4 February 2023.
https://orthomolecular.activehosted.com/index

Chapter 18: Photodynamic therapy

1. Johnstone D, Moro C, Stone J, et al. Turning On Lights to Stop Neurodegeneration: The Potential of Near Infrared Light Therapy in Alzheimer's and Parkinson's Disease. Front Neurosci 2015; 9: 500. www.ncbi.nlm.nih.gov/pmc/articles/PMC4707222/
2. Liang HL, Whelan HT, Eells JT, Wong-Riley MTT. Near-infrared light via light-emitting diode treatment is therapeutic against rotenone- and 1-methyl-4-phenylpyridinium ion-induced neurotoxicity. *Neuroscience* 2008; 153(4): 963-974. www.sciencedirect.com/science/article/abs/pii/S0306452208004065
3. Ying R, Liang HL, Whelan HT, Eells JT, Wong-Riley MTT. Pretreatment with near-infrared light via light-emitting diode provides added benefit against rotenone- and MPP+-induced neurotoxicity. *Brain Research* 2008; 1243: 167-173. doi: 10.1016/j.brainres.2008.09.057 www.sciencedirect.com/science/article/abs/pii/S0006899308023354
4. Quirk BJ, Torbey M, Buchmann E, et al. Near-infrared photobiomodulation in an animal model of traumatic brain injury: improvements at the behavioral and biochemical levels. *Photomed Laser Surg* 2012; 30(9): 5239. doi: 10.1089/pho.2012.3261 https://pubmed.ncbi.nlm.nih.gov/22793787/
5. Trimmer PA, Schwartz KM, Borland MK, et al. Reduced axonal transport in Parkinson's disease cybrid neurites is restored by light therapy. *Mol Neurodegener* 2009; 4: 26. doi: 10.1186/1750-1326-4-26 https://pubmed.ncbi.nlm.nih.gov/19534794/
6. Purushothuman S, Nandasena C, Johnstone DM, et al. The impact of near-infrared light on dopaminergic cell survival in a transgenic mouse model of parkinsonism. *Brain Res* 2013; 1535: 61-70. doi: 10.1016/j.brainres.2013.08.047 https://pubmed.ncbi.nlm.nih.gov/23998985/
7. Liebert A, Bicknell B, Laakso E-L, et al. Improvements in clinical signs of Parkinson's disease using photobiomodulation: a prospective proof-of-concept study. *BMC Neurol* 2021; 21(1): 256. doi: 10.1186/s12883-021-02248-y https://pubmed.ncbi.nlm.nih.gov/34215216/
8. Mythri RB, Bharath MMS. Curcumin: a potential neuroprotective agent in Parkinson's disease. *Curr Pharm Des* 2012; 18(1): 91-99. https://pubmed.ncbi.nlm.nih.gov/22211691/
9. Costantini A, Pala MI, Compagnoni L, Colangeli M. High-dose thiamine as initial treatment for Parkinson's disease. *BMJ Case Rep* 2013; 2013: bcr2013009289. doi: 10.1136/bcr-2013-009289 https://pubmed.ncbi.nlm.nih.gov/23986125/
10. Costantini A, Pala MI, Grossi E, et al. Long-Term Treatment with High-Dose Thiamine in Parkinson Disease: An Open-Label Pilot Study. *J Altern Complement Med* 2015; 21(12): 740-747. doi: 10.1089/acm.2014.0353 https://pubmed.ncbi.nlm.nih.gov/26505466/
11. Salehpour F, Khademi M, Hamblin MR. Photobiomodulation Therapy for Dementia: A Systematic Review of Pre-Clinical and Clinical Studies. *J Alzheimers Dis* 2021; 83(4): 1431-1452. doi: 10.3233/JAD-210029 https://pubmed.ncbi.nlm.nih.gov/33935090/

12. Longo MGF, Tan CO, Chan S-T, et al. Effect of Transcranial Low-Level Light Therapy vs Sham Therapy Among Patients With Moderate Traumatic Brain Injury: A Randomized Clinical Trial. *JAMA Netw Open* 2020; 3(9): e2017337. doi: 10.1001/jamanetworkopen.2020.17337 https://pubmed.ncbi.nlm.nih.gov/32926117/
13. Leisman G, Machado C, Machado Y, Chinchilla-Acosta M. Effects of Low-Level Laser Therapy in Autism Spectrum Disorder. *Adv Exp Med Biol* 2018; 1116: 111-130. doi: 10.1007/5584_2018_234. https://pubmed.ncbi.nlm.nih.gov/29956199/
14. Han Q, Lau JW, Do TC, Zhang Z, Xing B. Near-Infrared Light Brightens Bacterial Disinfection: Recent Progress and Perspectives. *ACS Appl Bio Mater* 2021; 4(5): 3937-3961. doi: 10.1021/acsabm.0c01341 https://pubmed.ncbi.nlm.nih.gov/35006816/
15. Lin C-C, Liu X-M, Peyton K, et al. Far Infrared Therapy Inhibits Vascular Endothelial Inflammation via the Induction of Heme Oxygenase-1. *Arteriosclerosis, Thrombosis, and Vascular Biology* 2008; 28(4): 739-745. www.ahajournals.org/doi/full/10.1161/atvbaha.107.160085
16. Pollack G. *Fourth Phase of Water: Beyond Solid, Liquid, and Vapor.* Ebner & Sons; 2013. www.amazon.co.uk/Fourth-Phase-Water-Beyond-Liquid/dp/0962689548
17. Cancer Research UK. Photodynamic therapy. Cancer Research UK. www.cancerresearchuk.org/about-cancer/treatment/other/photodynamic-therapy-PDT
18. Dos Santos AF, Terra LF, Wailemann RAM, et al. Methylene blue photodynamic therapy induces selective and massive cell death in human breast cancer cells. *BMC Cancer* 2017; 17(1): 194. doi: 10.1186/s12885-017-3179-7 https://pubmed.ncbi.nlm.nih.gov/28298203/

Chapter 19: Reprogramming the immune system with micro-immunotherapy

1. Naviaux R. Metabolic features of the cell danger response. *Mitochondrion* 2014; 16: 7-17. https://pubmed.ncbi.nlm.nih.gov/23981537/
2. Chen T, Song J, Liu H, et al. Positive Epstein-Barr virus detection in corona virus disease 2019 (COVID-19) patients. Research Square, www.researchsquare.com/article/rs-21580/v1
3. Gold J, Okyay RA, Licht WE, Hurley DJ. Investigation of Long COVID Prevalence and Its Relationship to Epstein-Barr Virus Reactivation. *Pathogens* 2021; 10(6): 763. doi: 10.3390/pathogens10060763. https://pubmed.ncbi.nlm.nih.gov/34204243/
4. Peluso MJ, Deveau T-M, Munter SE, et al. Impact of Pre-Existing Chronic Viral Infection and Reactivation on the Development of Long COVID. *Journal of Clinical Investigation*. 2023; 133(3): e163669. doi: 10.1172/JCI163669.
5. Micro-immunotherapy. *International Medical Experience* www.micro-immunotherapy.com/what-is-micro-immunotherapy/scientific-papers/ (accessed 23 October 2023)

Chapter 20: Reducing the infectious load

1. Burakgazi AZ. Lyme disease – induced polyradiculopathy mimicking amyotrophic lateral sclerosis. *International Journal of Neuroscience* 2014; 124(11): 859-862. doi: 10.3109/00207454.2013.879582
2. Myhill S. Valacyclovir in the treatment of post viral fatigue syndrome. September 2022. https://drmyhill.co.uk/wiki/Valacyclovir_in_the_treatment_of_post_viral_fatigue_syndrome
3. Langley GJ. The difficulties in diagnosis and treatment of hepatic abscess. *Br Med J* 1921; 2(3182): 1073–1074. www.ncbi.nlm.nih.gov/pmc/articles/PMC2339657/pdf/brmedj06827-0015.pdf

Chapter 21: The emotional holes in the energy bucket

1. Watts ME, Pocock R, Claudianos C. Brain Energy and Oxygen Metabolism: Emerging Role in Normal Function and Disease. *Front Mol Neurosci* 2018; 11: 216. doi: 10.3389/fnmol.2018.00216 www.ncbi.nlm.nih.gov/pmc/articles/PMC6023993
2. Davies J. *Cracked: Why Psychiatry is Doing More Harm Than Good.* Icon Books; 2013. www.amazon.co.uk/Cracked-Psychiatry-Doing-More-Harm/dp/1848315562

Chapter 22: The emotional hole in the energy bucket

1. *The Diagnostic and Statistical Manual of Mental Disorders, Fifth Edition* (DSM-5-TR). American Psychiatric Association Publishing. www.appi.org/products/dsm
2. Gerahty K, Jason L, Sunnquist M, et al. The 'cognitive behavioural model' of chronic fatigue syndrome: Critique of a flawed model. *Health Psychol Open* 2019; 6(1): 2055102919838907. doi: 10.1177/2055102919838907
3. National Institute for Health and Care Excellence. Myalgic encephalomyelitis (or encephalopathy)/chronic fatigue syndrome: diagnosis and management: NICE guideline [NG206]. 29 October 2021 www.nice.org.uk/guidance/ng206
4. Lyons L. The Post's New Yorker: Quote Page. *The Washington Post* 12 May 1937.
5. Plowden S. F. Scott Fitzgerald and literary synesthesia: The heightening of mood, moment, and ambiguity. www.proquest.com/openview/16450992339aa93d28cc25b68ae3e6fd/1.pdf
6. Floyd T. Your name tastes like purple. www.nbcnews.com/health/body-odd/your-name-tastes-purple-flna1c6437425

Chapter 23: The politics of CFS and ME

1. Laucks P, Salzman GA. The Dangers of Vaping. *Mo Med* 2020; 117(2): 159–164. www.ncbi.nlm.nih.gov/pmc/articles/PMC7144697/ PMID: 32308243
2. National Institutes of Health. NIH-funded studies show damaging effects of vaping, smoking on blood vessels. NIH News Release 26 October 2022. www.nih.gov/news-events/news-releases/nih-funded-studies-show-damaging-effects-vaping-smoking-blood-vessels (Accessed 20 August 2023)
3. National Institutes of Health. The Risks of Vaping. *News in Health* May 2020. https://newsinhealth.nih.gov/2020/05/risks-vaping (Accessed 20 August 2023)

4a. OpenVAERS www.openvaers.com

4b. OpenVAERS - Analysis of adverse effects on children www.openvaers.com/covid-data/child-summaries

4c. UK Freedom Project - Yellow Card Analysis https://ukfreedomproject.org/covid-19-vaccines-yellow-card-analysis/

4d. Dr Mark Trozzi Website https://drtrozzi.org/2023/09/28/1000-peer-reviewed-articles-on-vaccine-injuries/

5. Gregory AE, Titball R, Williamson D. Vaccine delivery using nanoparticles. *Front Cell Infect Microbiol* 2013; 3: 13. doi: 10.3389/fcimb.2013.00013 www.ncbi.nlm.nih.gov/pmc/articles/PMC3607064/
6. Hooper E. *The River: A journey to the source of HIV and AIDS.* Little, Brown and Company; 2000. https://www.amazon.co.uk/River-Journey-Source-HIV-AIDS/dp/0316371378/
7. Heckenlively K, Mikovits J. *Plague: One scientist's intrepid search for the truth about human retroviruses and ME/CFS, autism and other diseases.* Skyhourse Publishing; 2017.
8. Seneff S. *Toxic Legacy: How the weedkiller glyphosate is destroying our health and environment.* Chelsea Green Publishing; 2023.
9. Guardian Letters: Improving air quality requires a little less conversation, a lot more action. *Guardian* 7 April 2017. www.theguardian.com/environment/2017/apr/07/improving-air-quality-requires-a-little-less-conversation-a-lot-more-action
10. van Steenis D. Written Evidence 2 in: *House of Commons Environmental Audit Committee Air quality: A follow up report Ninth Report of Session 2010–12* Ev w 3; 9 November 2021. https://publications.parliament.uk/pa/cm201012/cmselect/cmenvaud/1024/1024vw.pdf (Accessed 20 August 2023)
11. Myhill S. Mercury – Toxicity of dental amalgam. www.drmyhill.co.uk/wiki/Mercury_-_Toxicity_of_Dental_Amalgam_-_Why_you_should_have_your_dental_amalgams_removed (Accessed 29 September 2023)
12. Ashford NA, Miller CS. *Chemical Exposures: Low levels, high stakes.* Second Edition.

John Wiley & Sons; 1998. http://tiltresearch.org/wp-content/uploads/sites/46/2019/03/Chemical_Exposures_Low_Levels_and_High_Stakes_2nd_Ed-min.pdf (accessed 23 October 2023)

13. Wright J. Chronic and occult carbon monoxide poisoning: we don't know what we're missing. *Emerg Med J* 2002; 19: 386–390. doi: 10.1136/emj.19.5.386
14. Bhuyan S. Effects of Microplastics on Fish and in Human Health. *Front Environ Sci* 16 March 2022; Sec Toxicology, Pollution and the Environment 2022; 10. doi: 10.3389/fenvs.2022.827289
15. Newby K. *Bitten: The secret history of Lyme disease and biological weapons.* Harper Wave; 2020. https://www.amazon.co.uk/Bitten-History-Disease-Biological-Weapons/dp/0062896288/
16. White PD, Goldsmith KA, Johnson AL, Potts L, Walwyn R, DeCesare et al. Comparison of adaptive pacing therapy, cognitive behaviour therapy, graded exercise therapy, and specialist medical care for chronic fatigue syndrome (PACE): a randomised trial. *Lancet* 2011; doi: 10.1016/S0140-6736(11)60096-2
17. https://informationrights.decisions.tribunals.gov.uk/DBFiles/Decision/i1854/Queen%20Mary%20University%20of%20London%20EA-2015-0269%20(12-8-16).PDF
18. Eliot Smith V. Tribunal orders release of PACE trial data (QMUL v the IC and Matthees). 16 August 2016. https://valerieeliotsmith.com/2016/08/16/tribunal-orders-release-of-pace-trial-data-qmul-v-the-ic-and-matthees/
19. Marks DF. Special Issue on the PACE Trial. *Journal of Health Psychology*. 2017; 22(9). doi: 10.1177/1359105317722370
20. Davis RW, Edwards JCW, Jason LA, et al. An open letter to Dr Richard Horton and The Lancet. *virology blog* 13 November 2015. www.virology.ws/2015/11/13/an-open-letter-to-dr-richard-horton-and-the-lancet/
21. Racaniello V. An open letter to The Lancet, again. *virology blog* 10 February 2016. www.virology.ws/2016/02/10/open-letter-lancet-again/
22. Tuller D. Trial by Error: An Open Letter to the Lancet, Two Years on. *virology blog* 19 June 2018. www.virology.ws/2018/06/19/trial-by-error-an-open-letter-to-the-lancet-two-years-on/

Appendix 2: Diet, detox and die-off (DDD) reactions

1. Nir G. Is the sky darkest just before dawn? Davidson Institute of Science Education 9 May 2017. https://davidson.weizmann.ac.il/en/online/askexpert/sky-darkest-just-dawn (accessed 6 June 2021)
2. Fulgoni VL, Keast DR, Lieberman HR. Trends in intake and sources of caffeine in the diets of US adults: 2001-2010. Am J Clin Nutr 2015; 101(5): 1081-1087.

doi: 10.3945/ajcn.113.080077; www.ncbi.nlm.nih.gov/pubmed/25832334
3. Cueto E. How old are caffeinated drinks? Bustle 16 September 2015. www.bustle.com/articles/110861-how-old-is-coffee-the-first-caffeinated-beverages-might-be-1200-years-old-so-heres-a (accessed 6 June 2021)

Appendix 3: Commonly used blood tests

1. Wannamethee G, et al. Low serum total cholesterol concentrations and mortality in middle aged British men. *Br Med J* 1995; 311(7002): 409-413. https://pubmed.ncbi.nlm.nih.gov/7640584/
2. Ravnskov U, et al. Lack of an association or an inverse association between low-density-lipoprotein cholesterol and mortality in the elderly: a systematic review. *Br Med J Open* 6(6): https://bmjopen.bmj.com/content/6/6/e010401
3. Honolulu Heart Program (HHP). https://biolincc.nhlbi.nih.gov/studies/hhp/
4. Borsche L, Glauner B, von Mendel J. Covid-19 mortality risk correlates inversely with vitamin D3 status, and a mortality rate close to zero could be theoretically achieved at 50 ng/mL 25(OH)D3: Results of a systematic review and meta-analysis. *Nutrients* 2021; 13(10): 3596. doi: 10.3390/nu13103596

Appendix 4: State welfare benefits – UK

1. Spring Budget 2023 factsheet – Disability White Paper. Gov.UK 15 March 2023. www.gov.uk/government/publications/spring-budget-2023-disability-white-paper-factsheet/spring-budget-2023-factsheet-disability-white-paper
2. National Institute for Health and Care Excellence (NICE). Myalgic encephalomyelitis (or encephalopathy)/chronic fatigue syndrome: diagnosis and management. NICE guideline [NG206] 29 October 2021. www.nice.org.uk/guidance/ng206
3. An ME Association Summary of the 2021 NICE Clinical Guideline for ME/CFS. Essential information from the new NICE Guideline. ME Association. December 2021. https://meassociation.org.uk/wp-content/uploads/NICE-Clinical-Guideline-on-MECFS-An-MEA-Summary-December-2021.pdf
4. ME Association. Employment and Support Allowance Work Capability Assessment review: Making it work for fluctuating conditions. April 2011. www.meassociation.org.uk/wp-content/uploads/Fluctuating_conditions_report_FINAL.pdf

Appendix 5: The Bell CFS Ability Scale

1.Wikipedia. David Sheffield Bell. https://en.wikipedia.org/wiki/David_Sheffield_Bell (accessed 23 October 2023)
2. Carruthers BM, van de Sande MI, De Meirleir KL, et al. Myalgic encephalomyelitis: International Consensus Criteria. *Journal of Internal Medicine* 2011; 270: 327-338. doi: 10.1111/j.1365-2796.2011.02428.x https://drmyhill.co.uk/drmyhill/images/4/4c/ME-INTERNATIONAL-CONCENSUS-CRITERIA.pdf

Useful Resources

Note: I am often asked by non-UK residents where they can obtain the supplements I recommend or their equivalents. I have tried to give some ideas below, but a key resource is my Facebook Group – see the links for Social Media Platforms below. Both of my Facebook groups run informal 'buddy schemes'; the idea is that a non-UK group member buddies up with a UK group member. The UK member orders the required supplement from within the UK and posts it to the non-UK Member and they sort out the money between themselves. Some long-lasting friendships have grown up in the 13 years that this scheme has been operational, resulting in at least one month-long holiday of a UK member at a US member's house!

Alternatively, non-UK members can use:

www.reship.com/services

They will ship from the UK to anywhere in the world.

General

My website: www.drmyhill.co.uk – contains 500+ pages of free, useful, health information, recently (2021-2023) fully updated.

My social media platforms for further support: https://drmyhill.co.uk/wiki/My_Social_Media_Presence (Facebook, 'X', YouTube, Instagram)

Patient-generated sources of support:
www.drmyhill.co.uk/wiki/CFS/ME_support_organisations

My books

On my website: www.salesatdrmyhill.co.uk/dr-myhills-books-10-c.asp

On the publisher's website: www.hammersmithbooks.co.uk (includes ebooks)

And from all online vendors, including Amazon.co.uk, Amazon.com, BooksEtc, Booktopia (Australia) and Chelsea Green (USA and Canada)

Sunshine Salt

www.salesatdrmyhill.co.uk/sunshine-salt-300-g-392-p.asp

Saltpipe

For use with Lugol's iodine (see below):

- www.salesatdrmyhill.co.uk/saltpipe---easy-saltpipe-by-cisca-523-p.asp
- www.amazon.com/Natural-Inhaler-Respiratory-Issues-Allergies/dp/B07B47X2MD
- Many other online shops and independent health food stores

Transdermal products

www.salesatdrmyhill.co.uk/transdermal-nutrients-12-c.asp

PatchAid Vitamin and Mineral patches: https://patchaid.com/collections/vitamin-and-mineral-patches-by-patchaid

The Basic and Mitochondrial packages

The Basic Package: www.salesatdrmyhill.co.uk/package---basic-package-new-starter-kit---4-items-hempiness-728-p.asp

The Mitochondrial Package: www.salesatdrmyhill.co.uk/package---mitochondrial-package-starter-kit--5-items-667-p.asp

For non-UK purchasers: As an example of some of these products and where they can be bought from non-UK sites:

- Amazon.com – D ribose: www.amazon.com/D-Ribose-High-Purity-Fine-Powder/dp/B07GHY8S88/

- Amazon.com – Acetyl L carnitine: www.amazon.com/NOW-Acetyl-L-Carnitine-750-Tablets/dp/B0013OQI6W/ref=sr_1_1
- B12 ampoules (German site): www.apohealth.de/collections/all/products/pascoe-vitamin-b12-depot-injektopas-1500-g-ampullen-10-st-ampullen

DMSO and methylene blue

For DMSO:

- www.salesatdrmyhill.co.uk/dmso-500ml-of-super-pure-synthesis-grade-dmso-x28-dimethyl-sulfoxide-x29-940-p.asp
- www.amazon.com/Pharma-DMSO-99-99-Absolutely-Odorless/dp/B01LBGIRMY/ref=sr_1_4
- Dr Moran's deodorised preparation: www.drmorans.com/products/dmso-dimethyl-sulfoxide

For methylene blue:

- www.salesatdrmyhill.co.uk/methylene-blue-powder---10g-plus-syringe-944-p.asp
- and from many more online sites

Vitamins, minerals and supplements – Suppliers

- UK – www.salesatdrmyhill.co.uk
- UK – www.biocare.co.uk
- UK – www.naturesbest.co.uk
- USA – www.swansonvitamins.com
- USA – www.puritan.com
- And numerous other good suppliers –Lamberts, Viridian Nutrition, Igennus, Now, Doctor's Best, Pure Health, Jarrow Formulas, Bulk (good for vitamin C), Healthy Origins, Nature's Way

Herbals – Suppliers

- UK – www.indigo-herbs.co.uk
- UK – www.hybridherbs.co.uk
- USA – www.mountainroseherbs.com

Sleep supplements – Suppliers

- Melatonin: Bioeva – go to www.biovea.com/uk/ and search for 'Melatonin' for a full list of their extensive DHEA products. Also, from their US site: www.biovea.com/US/productlist/results?KW=melatonin
- Nytol: High Street chemists – for example, https://lloydspharmacy.com/collections/nytol and Amazon: www.amazon.com/Nytol-Nighttime-Sleep-Aid-Caplets-32/dp/B000052YEN
- Nytol Herbal: www.salesatdrmyhill.co.uk/nytol-herbal-30-tablets-175-p.asp
- Valerian: supplement and herbal suppliers as above – for example, www.naturesbest.co.uk/herbs-spices/valerian/valerian-tablets/
- Kava kava: www.amazon.com/kava/s?k=kava+kava and many other online suppliers: search for 'kava kava'

Thyroid glandulars – Suppliers

- Procepts Nutrition Metavive I, II, III, IV (UK product): www.the-natural-choice.co.uk/Endocrine-Thyroid-Adrenals.html
- Metavive I (porcine thyroid complex 40 mg) – delivers 15 mg porcine glandular
- Metavive II (porcine thyroid complex 80 mg) – delivers 30 mg porcine glandular
- Metavive III (bovine thyroid complex 40 mg) delivers 15 mg bovine glandular
- Metavive IV (bovine thyroid complex 80 mg) delivers 30 mg bovine glandular

Also see:

- www.salesatdrmyhill.co.uk/metavive-i----180-capsules-547-p.asp
- www.salesatdrmyhill.co.uk/metavive-ii---90-capsules-549-p.asp
- Ancestral Supplements Grassfed Beef Thyroid: www.ancestralsupplements.com
- Dr. Ron's Ultra-Pure Thyroid With Liver: www.drrons.com
- Forefront Health Raw Desiccated Thyroid: www.forefronthealth.com
- Natural Sources Raw Thyroid: www.vitacost.com
- Nutri-Meds Desiccated Thyroid: www.nutri-meds.com

Adrenal supplements – Suppliers

Pregnenolone:

- www.salesatdrmyhill.co.uk/pregnenolone-by-swansons---50-mg---60-capsules-793-p.asp – 50 mg capsule size

- https://uk.iherb.com/pr/life-extension-pregnenolone-50-mg-100-capsules/4380 – 50 mg capsule size
- www.dolphinfitness.co.uk/en/swanson-pregnenolone-25mg-60-capsules/325050 – 25 mg capsule size
- (US site): www.lifeextension.com/vitamins-supplements/item00700/pregnenolone

DHEA:

- Bioeva: www.biovea.com/uk/ and search 'DHEA' for a full list of their extensive DHEA products.
- Piping Rock: https://gb.pipingrock.com/v2/dhea
- Life Extension: www.lifeextension.com/search#q=dhea&t=coveo4A2453FD

Bovine glandulars:

- www.dolphinfitness.co.uk/en/swanson-adrenal-glandular-60-capsules/200072
- www.the-natural-choice.co.uk/Endocrine-Thyroid-Adrenals.html
- (US site): www.gembrahealth.com

Iodine supplements – Suppliers

- Lugol's Iodine 15%: www.salesdrmyhill.co.uk/lugols-iodine-15-463.p.asp and https://essentialminerals.co.uk/15-lugols-iodine/ and many other suppliers
- Lugol's Iodine 12%: www.amazon.co.uk/Iodine-12-Lugols-Solution-30ml/dp/B07KTB3S7B/ and www.healthleadsuk.com/lugols-iodine-solution-12-percent.html and many other suppliers.
- Iodoral (12.5 mg): www.amazon.co.uk/Iodoral-12-5-mg-180-tablets/dp/B000X843VG/ and www.desertcart.co.uk/products/48162034-iodoral-12-5-mg-180-tablets and many other suppliers
- Betadine: Povidone-Iodine Ointment – www.salesatdrmyhill.co.uk/betadine---povidone-iodine-ointment-20g-758-p.asp and other suppliers
- Non-UK readers: You may not be able to obtain the 12% or 15% strength Lugol's Iodine. You can buy 2% strength and scale up the doses accordingly from: www.amazon.com/EPOTHEX-Solution-Dropper-Contains-Potassium/dp/B0CBCXL1GD/ref=sr_1_1_sspa

Testing

- For a full list of laboratories see 'Natural Health Worldwide': https://naturalhealthworldwide.com/lab-tests/
- No practitioner referral is needed for these:
  - https://medichecks.com
  - https://smartnutrition.co.uk/
- These laboratories require a practitioner referral:
  - www.gdx.net
  - www.doctorsdata.com
  - www.tdlpathology.com
  - https://aonm.org – This is the UK distributor of www.arminlabs.com/en – very useful for tests of infections.
- Comprehensive stool test: https://smartnutrition.co.uk/digestion/ digestive-testing/ gi-effects-comprehensive-stool-test/
- Adrenal stress test: https://smartnutrition.co.uk/health-tests/adrenal-stress-test
- DMSA for toxic metal chelation: From Smart Nutrition at £118.00 (at time of going to press) for the test plus cost of DMSA: https://smartnutrition.co.uk/health-tests/toxic-heavy-metals/
- Non-UK readers can rest assured that their respective countries will have private labs that provide equivalent tests.

Natural Health Worldwide

This support network now includes 18 medical doctors (as of November 2023), 155 Qualified Health Professionals and 37 Experienced Patients.

- https://naturalhealthworldwide.com/category/practitioners/medical-doctor/
- https://naturalhealthworldwide.com/category/practitioners/qualified-health-practitioner/
- https://naturalhealthworldwide.com/category/practitioners/experienced-patient/

There are also lists of laboratories and mobile phlebotomists:

- https://naturalhealthworldwide.com/lab-tests/
- https://naturalhealthworldwide.com/mobile-phlebotomists/

Thermometers

FIR (far infrared) skin thermometers can be obtained from many suppliers, including:

- www.amazon.co.uk/Thermometer-Femometer-Digital-Forehead-Accurate/dp/B0865RL4PH/ref=sr_1_2_sspa
- www.boots.com/boots-non-contact-thermometer-10192058
- US site: www.amazon.com/EPOTHEX-Solution-Dropper-Contains-Potassium/dp/B0CBCXL1GD/

For a full range of thermometers:

- www.boots.com/baby-child/nursery-furniture/thermometers
- Digital: www.amazon.com/Vicks-SpeedRead-Digital-Thermometer-V912US/dp/B000GRXHIE/

Urine ketostix and urine infection products

- Ketostix:
  - www.salesatdrmyhill.co.uk/ketostix-50-test-strips-317-p.asp
  - www.amazon.com/Ketostix-Reagent-Strips-BOX-EACH/dp/B007AZ686I/
- D-Mannose:
  - www.salesatdrmyhill.co.uk/d-mannose-capsules---500-mg---120-veg-capsules-583-p.asp
  - www.salesatdrmyhill.co.uk/d-mannose-powder---85-g-99-p.asp
  - www.amazon.com/D-Mannose-500-Now-Foods-VCaps/dp/B0768FVKFJ/
- Potassium citrate:
  - Effervescent tablets (brand Effercitrate): take 2 tablets dissolved into a whole glass of water, up to 3 times a day
  - Liquid medicine (brand Cymaclear): take 2 x 5-ml spoonfuls, stirred into a whole glassful of water, to 3 doses a day
  - Sachets (brand Cystopurin): empty the contents of 1 sachet into a whole glassful of water and stir well before drinking, 3 times daily
  - US: www.amazon.com/Potassium-Citrate-Powder-Herbal-Effects/dp/B0CGWZ8THL/ref=sr_1_7
  - And many other online suppliers

Ketone breath meters

There are many good types – read the reviews online.

Read this article for reviews of seven such meters: https://bodyketosis.com/ketone-breath-analyzer/

Many of my Facebook Group members use this device: www.amazon.co.uk/dp/B07VJMNMCD/ref=as_li_ss_tl

US (Amazon): www.amazon.com/Portable-Digital-Analyzer-Replaceable-Mouthpieces/dp/B0BP133WYT/

FIR (far infrared) products

- Get Fitt: www.get-fitt.com
- Firzone:
  - www.firzone.co.uk/portable-infrared-sauna-standard.html
  - www.firzone.co.uk/single-zone-sauna-blanket.html
- For activating DMSO and methylene blue:
  - www.amazon.co.uk/Nebula-LED-Light-Therapy-Belt/dp/B0BMQW39BS/
- FIR blanket: www.amazon.com/Portable-Digital-Analyzer-Replaceable-Mouthpieces/dp/B0BP133WYT/
- LED light therapy belt: www.amazon.com/Scienlodic-Light-Therapy-Belt-Body/dp/B0C39W32KC/

Vitamin C urine test strips

These are readily available online – for example, see:

www.amazon.co.uk/Vitamin-Strips-Urine-Analysis-VitaChek-C/dp/B00K2265JQ

www.amazon.com/Ascorbic-Acid-Vitamin-Food-Strip/dp/B07G7HCYX9/

Food suppliers

- Vegan cheese: Bute Island (www.buteisland.com) for vegan cheese
- Sauerkraut: Goodness Direct (www.goodnessdirect.co.uk)
- Grace Coconut Milk: from my website (www.salesatdrmyhill.co.uk/coconut-milk-1-litre-grace-pre¬mium-thai-335-p.asp) and other good food sites)

- Organic golden linseed: Many of the Dr Myhill Facebook Group members use Suma Organic Golden Linseed (www.amazon.co.uk/Suma-Prepacks-Organic-Linseed-Golden/dp/B01061U62Y/ref=sr_1_6) and there are many other good suppliers
- Organic vegetable box delivery: www.abelandcole.co.uk or look for a local farm supplier

Micro-immunotherapy

www.micro-immunotherapy.com

Advice on how to garden organically

Garden Organic: Formerly known as Henry Doubleday Research Association, for advice on how to garden organically whether your garden is large or small go to: www.gardenorganic.org.uk/

Index

Note the following terms: A, Appendix; *n*, footnote.

Note the following terms: A, Appendix; *n*, footnote.

Index

Note the following terms: A, Appendix; *n*, footnote.

Note the following terms: A, Appendix; *n*, footnote.

Note the following terms: A, Appendix; *n*, footnote.